It Matters Totally

Healing Food Addiction with
A Course in Miracles

MARIELLE SCHOOL AND LISA NATOLI

authorHOUSE®

I can think of. What I care about now is taking care of my beautiful self just as I do my darling daughter. It is effortless to care for her and now I'm finding immense pleasure in caring for myself.

Awesome work ladies!
xoxoxoxoxoxoxo
Suzanne

————————————————————————

I love *It Matters Totally*! I didn't think I needed it because I don't have a weight problem, but I figured it couldn't hurt. So I read the first entry, wrote a commitment letter, listened to the audio, and I realize now how much this program can help me. I am not a food addict and not overweight, but I don't take care of myself, and this became apparent to me in thinking about today's topic. Thanks for all your good work girls!

Carrie

————————————————————————

Dear Marielle & Lisa,

The two of you are marvelous for creating *It Matters Totally*. Wow! This 40 day program is the best thing that has ever happened to me. My God, has it opened my eyes! Do I ask for help? Am I my own best friend? Do I play everyday? And all the other wonderful ideas the program presents to let me understand that my eating addiction DID NOT JUST HAPPEN.

I am comforted by Marielle's story. If she hadn't gone down this path before us, I don't think I would be so confident it will work. But I know it will work, because it *is* working. I see changes in me already. Thank you so much for your love! Wishing you a joyous day,

Tery

————————————————————————

This program is amazing! Before I started, I was in so much pain - I could hardly walk. When I went through a simple meditation and offered my gifts to God at the altar, my back and leg felt almost 100%! It truly was a miracle! Now I don't expect huge miracles like that all the time, but it sure is amazing. I am new to *A Course in Miracles* and I am grateful to have you helping and guiding me through this journey.

God Bless, Linda

———————————————————

It Matters Totally is absolutely fabulous! Your daily messages are so inspiring. I feel like a kid that wants to try EVERYTHING. And it is hilariously FUN. I have really no time for problems - I'm so occupied with experimenting and seeing things differently! I am happy and I feel alive!!!

Love,
Jeannine

———————————————————

Dear Lisa & Marielle,

I am grateful for you two beauties. This 40 day course is incredible! Wow! It surpasses all expectations! You are doing a spectacular job guiding us to know our perfection.

Marisa

———————————————————

Hi Marielle & Lisa,

I am experiencing miracles in my life! What astonishes me the most is when I've got my attention on being helpful and not worrying about what others think of me, or how I look, or if I said the right thing and so on, I get so many compliments from people! And the compliments are completely opposite from how I generally feel about myself. I am seeing things differently. Thanks girls!

Lori

This morning I sat in my space. I spent time with my journal. It was lovely. It was just for me and just for the pure joy. Blossoming trees outside the window. I woke up thinking: "This is my day and I dedicate it to joy." Wow! I never had a thought like that before! What a great feeling allowing this gift to myself!!! I was nice to myself. It was a little scary. Am I really allowed to have fun for two days in a row? For 40 days?? Wow.
Thank you!!!!
I love you!!!!

Caroline

———————————————————————

This topic of dealing with limitations is the story of my life! My life has totally been about not finishing ANYTHING I start. It is about not even taking the first step because I'm afraid... or I don't want to do the work to get the goal I have in my mind. Working with this topic will be KEY for me. And I NEVER, ever looked at it... knew it was even there until I read this.

This 40-day program really rocks my boat. I never thought about miracles and change. Lisa, you wrote: "In order for it to be a miracle, it means that something unexpected and spontaneous would occur for you."

Whammo! That really got my attention! Guess what I have been fearing MOST? That something unexpected and spontaneous would occur for me. I might lose control. But now I'm laughing! I love it!!!! Bring it on!

Thanks so much for this program.

xoxo
Jenna

it matters Totally

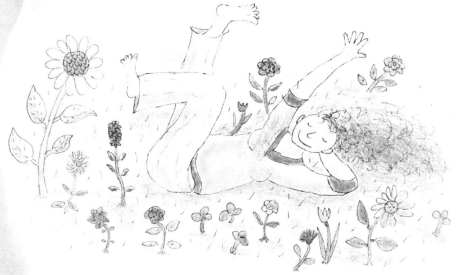

Healing food addiction with A Course in Miracles

Marielle School
and Lisa Natoli

AuthorHouse™
1663 Liberty Drive
Bloomington, IN 47403
www.authorhouse.com
Phone: 1-800-839-8640

First published by AuthorHouse 2/24/2010

ISBN: 978-1-4490-6618-5 (sc)

Library of Congress Control Number: 2009913896

Printed in the United States of America
Bloomington, Indiana

This book is printed on acid-free paper.

Editorial Supervision: Karyn Aldin
Cover Design: Sherri Nestorowich
Author Photograph: Rob Sötemann
Cover/Back Illustration & Interior Illustrations: Marielle School

Grateful acknowledgement to Jesus and A Course in Miracles.
Quotes noted as "ACIM" are from A Course in Miracles, published by the Foundation for
Inner Peace.
Quotes noted as "Urtext" are from the original manuscript of A Course in Miracles
called the "Urtext." For more information: http://courseinmiracles.com

Abraham-Hicks opening quote: Excerpted from an Abraham-Hicks workshop in Tampa,
FL on Saturday, December 6th, 2003 #234
For more information: http://www.abraham-hicks.com

This book is dedicated to Share Murphy, who encouraged us to publish *"It Matters Totally"* as a book.

You're a Superstar!

We are forever grateful for your enthusiasm and trust. You're a true inspiration.

We also dedicate this book to all the beautiful people in the world who, just like us, need the reminder that there is help and love available with this often devastating disease.

This is what we stand for.

And finally, we are grateful to everyone that participated in our original online program. We were just getting our feet wet, wandering around in unchartered territory. You stood right there with us, every step of the way, our mighty companions! Your dedication, feedback, questions and comments were invaluable and stay with us as the foundation of this program.

Thank you.

Table of Contents

"The purpose of these exercises is to train the mind to a different perception of everyone and everything in the world."

– A Course in Miracles

"You're always getting a perfect vibrational match to what you predominantly give your attention to. But you've got to make the best of it. You've got to vibrate slightly different from where you are if you are going to improve where you are. You can't keep taking score of where your business is or your relationship is, or your body is, without continuing to create it as it is. To make improvement, you've got to reach for a different thought."

-Abraham-Hicks (Jerry & Esther Hicks)
http://www.abraham-hicks.com

Preface by Lisa Natoli

It Matters Totally began as conversations at Starbucks. Marielle and I have been friends since 2001 when we met at an academy for ministers in Wisconsin. She's from Holland and I'm from New Hampshire. When I first met her, she was mostly depressed, angry, tired, overweight, and she cried a lot. She had moments when her true creative child would burst through and then she would be playful, beautiful, spontaneous, generous and happy. But mostly, she was depressed. When I looked at her, it was like looking at someone in a black cloud.

I was overweight but I didn't call it a food addiction. I wasn't bulimic or anorexic, though I did spend almost all my time thinking about food. I spent my days shopping for food, planning meals, and eating. I ate when I was bored, happy, anxious, joyful, depressed and excited. I ate for pleasure, for fun, to relieve stress and to feel comfort. Food to me was exciting. I liked thinking about it and talking about it. When I wasn't eating or cooking, I was searching the internet for diets and ways to lose weight. Looking back, it's easy to see I was obsessed and addicted. I joined chat groups for support. I bought inspirational books to help me transform my life. I was forever on the latest diet: vegan, raw vegan, protein shakes, no sugar, no carbs. I was constantly in the supermarket. My days revolved around the next meal. I would buy clothes that were too small for me in the hopes that someday I would be fabulously gorgeous and my life would begin. I lived mostly in fantasy. I thought all this was normal since almost everyone with whom I interacted was obsessed with food also. I really didn't think I had an addiction problem. I simply thought life would be better if I lost weight.

Then life took Marielle and I in different directions. I moved to New York and Marielle got pregnant and we didn't see each other for about a year.

When I saw Marielle next, she was completely transformed. She had a brand new gorgeous little baby girl named Julia along with a brand new body. She was happy with the energy of a teenager. She was vibrant and beautiful. She was alive and sparkling. Here was a girl who had been plagued by a life-long food addiction transformed into someone I could scarcely recognize. What was she eating?? I wanted to know. She said she was eating everything she wanted. There was no diet. In fact, she said she was eating more than ever before in her life. I kept thinking, "Yeah, right. Liar. Come on. Tell me what you're eating. What did you do? I'm your friend."

She kept saying "I didn't do anything" which I felt was the biggest lie in the world. She must have done something! I hounded her for answers. But she continued to tell me again and again she didn't do anything. I kept probing. It was like being a detective searching for clues, or an archaeologist digging for gold. I started observing her. I followed her around, watching her eating patterns. I was determined to find out what she was eating, and was shocked to find that she DID eat everything she wanted. Pasta, cheese, chocolate, fruits, vegetables, coffee, cookies. She didn't deprive herself in any way. So, how the hell did she get that body and all that joy?

Finally she gave me an answer: "Extreme Self-Care."

In a nutshell, Marielle made a decision to give up her addiction and to start being happy. She gave up all her pills, diets and groups. She stopped dieting. She said, simply: "I JUST WANT TO BE HAPPY."

She started living her life. She started taking care of herself. She started being nice to herself. She stopped attacking herself. She nurtured herself like a newborn baby. She ate whatever she wanted. There were no rules. Initially, she gained tons of weight. She didn't care. She made a decision she was "done with dieting", and she was sticking with it. She said she would prefer to be 300 pounds than to be trapped in the hell of addiction.

And then a curious thing started to happen: her body began to transform. As she became more peaceful and happy, her body started to change.

As she continued to do the work on her mind, her body naturally returned to its natural perfect state, without dieting.

She was healed from food addiction as she made a decision to stop sabotaging herself with endless diets. Instead of hating her body, she began loving her Self. She played, she danced, she spent time in nature, she bought clothes that fit her, and she started living her life instead of waiting for some future magical moment. That's the big secret.

I kept digging. I was relentless. I wanted more details. I wanted specifics. TELL ME MORE. I started taking notes. I wrote down everything Marielle said and I began to see that she absolutely DID do something to heal herself of food addiction, just that it had nothing at all to do with food.

She talked and I wrote. I questioned and she answered. This book is based on her ideas which I had to extract from her like a dentist pulling teeth (without being quite so painful as most of our interactions were at Starbucks over cake and coffee). It's not that she was trying to hide anything, but rather, that the "process" of transformation happened to her so naturally and so simply that she really didn't think there was anything to say on the subject. As far as she was concerned, one day she was a food addict and the next day... she was not.

This program is not about food at all. There's no diet. It's 40 days of 40 topics designed to catapult you into a new space where there is only love. It was created to overcome obstacles, stumbling blocks and addiction. It's about nurturing, purification and remembering that you are a precious child of God. It's about finding your passion and purpose.

And the name "*It Matters Totally*"? We have found that a lot of food addicts have feelings of hopelessness along with a feeling of resignation that "nothing matters." We wanted to give a reminder that *"It Matters Totally."* Your life matters totally. You matter totally. What you do matters totally.

That's the book you are now holding in your hands. *It Matters Totally.* You Matter Totally. If you have struggled with food addiction, get ready for big changes!

We cover 40 topics in 40 days to help you emerge from limitations and obstacles that have been keeping you from being your most vibrant, gorgeous self.

I am grateful to Marielle for sharing her experience of healing and transformation with me. I am happy to know there is a solution and that I don't have to suffer anymore waiting for my life to begin. And now with this book, neither do you!

Love,

Lisa

Introduction by Marielle School

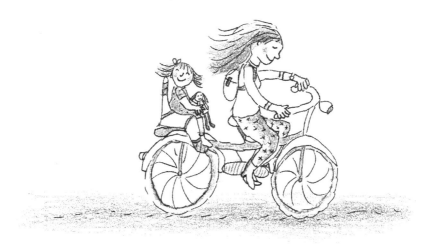

This is my story of food addiction. This is also a story of Grace, and my healing, which I hope now to extend in love to you.

Retracing my story, remembering the seductive nature of this addiction, the words that come to me are "it was not easy." Yet I see now how every step into myself was heavily supported by the universe, and in that sense, miraculous. My "way" was to take tiny little steps, learning to listen to myself, to trust, and to abandon my fear. Needless to say, it took me a while.

I feel very relieved now to be in a space of complete openness... to feel so relaxed about myself and know my life is really blessed. Life now is full of joy, and I do all the fun things that I want to!

I am no longer able to stay in negative situations or emotions for very long at all.

It is such a privilege to share this transformation with you, because I know if I can be healed of food addiction, anybody can. The key is that you are free. I can look at you in a light, one that you have perhaps forgotten, that will bring you great joy. It is my honor to help you to see yourself anew, to remember who you *really* are.

All you need is the commitment to get to know yourself, and to hold yourself like I did.

I have so much joy now just being myself because I dropped the compulsion to be perfect. I feel like all the separate parts in me are showing up, presenting themselves to me, unafraid to be "seen" now. In that, I am healed.

I can see now that in my life I always was surrounded with beautiful and helpful people and that the only thing that was missing was ME. It was super exciting to develop a relationship with that girl... with "me"!

Over the course of my healing, I turned from an old looking 20 year old to a young looking 40 year old. I found out that I still am very playful and that I have a great ability to have fun and to enjoy little things. I literally received myself and I learned to be consistent in this; to open to my own embrace. I learned to stay connected with my own flow. I learned a willingness to support myself in everything.

That blessed time came for me in which I never again would fall back into the food addiction anymore. I had become completely free from the obsession that hunted *and* haunted me for such a big part of my life. It felt almost "suddenly"! I had come to recognize myself in a new light. Yet, in reviewing and remembering, the story seems to have been one of challenge, determination, and victory – culminating in a resurrection of sorts.

It is hard to imagine it now. Yet here, following, I share a short summary of it with you.

Basically I abandoned myself from a very young age.

I felt like I was not "right" - the way I was - and that I needed to be different. I started to observe other people to see what was required from me and how I should behave and "be". This became an all consuming habit.

I was very hard on myself and I remember that I criticized even the way I peeled peanuts when I was 7. I felt very insecure. At school, I imitated and copied the other children. It was almost like I was just an observer. Still I was also a very playful child, and that literally saved me.

When I was at home I disappeared into beautiful secret worlds. In there, I was a fairy or a circus acrobat, and I was happy and free.

Often, too, I was found drawing and painting. Art made me very happy. Everything was good in my own made up world. I also intensely enjoyed family gatherings and the change of seasons. I remember embracing the cold air, walking to school, taking my time. And I remember enjoying quiet moments in the school yards before the other kids arrived.

I loved animals and nature. I loved just running around and climbing trees. I felt so happy as a child, just "being". But in relationship with other people – as with my classmates - I felt like I was nothing.

It was like I could not really be, in any real sense, happy with myself. I was completely insecure about "me"; but in my own world I was queen of the castle.

I started to have friendships with younger children who adored my world. And I lost touch with *me* in the world. And then, when I turned 12, a particularly difficult time came.

I did not want to grow up, and I felt especially insecure about my changing body. At school, the boys teased me and I felt so ugly and ashamed with myself and my looks. I was very shy. I felt not wanted.

Food became the answer to my run from myself, and the suppression of any natural impulse. I needed it to numb my feelings of hopelessness and my intense fear of rejection. I felt a constant shame about myself, and I could not stand the intensity of my loneliness.

There were times where I withheld treats from myself, and I would collect all the candy that I received in a big jar. Then I would fantasize about giving a party and sharing it with my school mates.

But suddenly I ate the whole jar of candy in one single serving. I was shocked and felt sick. I decided I was not to be trusted at any time.

I never realized that I shared my life with others. Even though I had a sister and both parents living with me, I mostly felt completely isolated. I never talked about my problems with food and life in general or my depression and my fears.

Through the years I had one friend that served as my role model and my savior. I copied her, and yet I tried to avoid her most of the time, to be alone in my food obsession.

Physically, when my teens came, I developed very quickly into a woman. I felt so much shame about it, and retreated more. Food helped me through my day.

I felt fat all the time and I tried to diet. It mostly did not work. I turned 18 and I moved out from my parents' house to a different city to study. Again I developed one friendship. But she was away during the weekends to be with her boyfriend, and I felt completely alone in the big student complex where I lived.

I started to have uncontrollable binges. I would literally eat everything I had, including food of my flat mates and the old bread that was meant for a pet rabbit. I was often so sick that I could not eat for 3 or 4 days.

One day my friend mentioned something about my "big cheeks", and I was completely shattered. I made a vow to eat as little as possible and to lose weight. And finally it worked.

I hardly had to eat anymore. And I was happy. This was my new purpose.

I decided to continue that way so that when I needed to eat a lot it would be okay. And I would not get fat. Continuing this way, I lost weight, and lots of it. I could not stop it anymore. I wanted to see all of my ribs, and I was so grateful not to have to face any fat anymore. From now on I was free from it. I did not need food anymore like other people. I felt purified and strong.

But the victory soon changed into fear when I recognized that I could not really eat any more. I was too afraid. Whenever I ate, I now had to walk or cycle long distances to make sure I would not get fat. My teeth got really bad, I was constantly cold, and I could not sleep very much anymore.

But still I felt content that I no longer had to get fat, and the little food that I still could eat meant the world to me. I felt really stuck, because I felt the contradiction all the time. I did not want to deal with a body anymore. It felt great to me to be so light and unattached. But at the same time I was always hungry and restless and depressed.

I ended up in a clinic to work on myself and to gain weight. I kept on struggling because I lived simply to be liked and loved by my psychiatrist, and I had no idea how to have a life of my own.

As soon as I left the clinic I lost all the weight that I gained there and I ended up all alone in a little apartment in a big city. I was 21 years old. I was weak and had developed a liver disease. I knew that I was killing myself, and that I had to make a commitment to life.

So I did. And after a year of isolation I moved to another city, and I started a performing arts school. But with that I started to lose my control over food again. It brought me straight back into the feelings of despair and loneliness that I experienced before I started my rigorous diet. I recognized that I had no control over food. I started to gain weight.

This brought me into a new aspect of my disease: purging. It was very addictive. At first I was so excited about it. I could get rid of the food, and I did not have to get fat! What a solution! But soon it became a nightmare. I would eat and throw up several times a day. It was impossible to break the cycle. The need to throw up became overwhelming. Afterwards my face would swell up, my throat would hurt, and I would feel completely weak. I would be dizzy and tremble, but I could not stop it. I kept it completely secret.

At this stage I asked for help again.

Finally I met people that had the same problems. I connected with God, and for the first time in my life, I did not feel alone. I found others that did all this crazy stuff with food. I felt, at last, that I could stop blaming myself for my crazy behavior.

Somehow I received the strength to stop purging. It made me gain weight very quickly and in three months I gained 70 pounds. It was shocking. I felt like a complete failure.

It took me another ten years to find out that this did not change my food addiction. I still felt fat, while simultaneously fighting against the desire to purge, as well as to be "clean" of the addiction. I could not touch the real me, the one that I had rejected so early in life.

During that time I went to a seminar with a woman who was running a clinic for people with anorexia in Canada. That was a revelation. Basically she showed me that all I needed to do was to give myself all the space I needed to be nourished, to respect myself, and to receive myself like a baby, in a whole new way. I needed to focus on me and my life.

Oh, did that seem impossible! But the seed was planted, although it needed a moment to sink in.

I still was very hard on myself and I tried so hard to fit in, "to give" what was asked from me, and to be truly helpful. I tried to be a "good girl", and to be an inspiration.

But I wasn't. I could not get myself out of the cycle of obsession with food. I was terrified to be myself. And I could not let myself be the most important thing in my life. It was completely alien not to focus on others anymore. I had to fall yet even more deeply. Into myself. I felt like a complete fool. Here I was all spiritual and gifted with so many tools to be happy. I had a great boyfriend, a nice apartment in Amsterdam, friends.

Yet I was so hungry inside, still just looking for an answer outside and a way to reject myself... a way to be someone else, and simultaneously, a new me.

Then I found *A Course in Miracles*. It totally shocked me. What was that!? It really touched me to the bone. I decided to learn more about it. I moved to the United States to attend a school that completely dedicated itself to this course.

It blew me away. I thought that I could just burn my bridges and leave myself behind. This was not true. This was not what forgiveness was and I did not see it.

So I still suffered a lot from lack of self-acceptance. I needed to understand the magic words, "Love myself, know myself, communicate with myself." But I had no idea how to do this.

It was a miracle that gave me my life back, honestly. I don't know how it started. It just appeared. Like a new era. Slowly, it just happened. I started a relationship with myself.

It was painful in the beginning. But I felt so happy with every little thing that I did for myself, that I realized that this was the key. It wasn't the focus on food or health or doing it right. It wasn't spiritual exercises, but simply the practice of learning to listen to myself.

Little steps. Little changes.

And soon the obsession with food fell away and I did not even think about it anymore. My body transformed into a whole new, beautiful shape. It all happened just as a by-product of my willingness to change my mind and to trust myself again. I found the ways to love myself and to learn to speak a new language with myself. The food continued to take care of itself. I became my own counselor, my own source of strength. I found out that there is no god outside of me, no relationship outside myself, nothing outside myself at all.

And that is where Lisa showed up in my life again; right there in the beginning of this new change. She helped me enormously to develop a friendship based on freedom, mutual respect and fun. She never saved me. She trusted my own saviorship. And she was there for me. I did not have to compete with her, or to make her feel good. I could be myself from the very start.

I adored her and it was kind of like summer even in the midst of winter, because there she was, all available and laughing and light-hearted. I completely flourished in that light. I felt that I found my purpose. I was in the beginning of my life and it was not graceful or elegant, but it was OK! Often it felt very uncomfortable and I felt lost. Yet somehow I had the willingness to get in there where I had never wanted to go before. I discovered right where there existed the true instruction for *my personal journey.*

There was no way around it, nor a more "civil" way to learn this.

At that point Lisa started to ask me about my healing with my food addiction and I shared it with her. She wanted a way to be reminded in those moments of forgetting. So we started to tape the story of healing, what I did, and how it happened. Lisa asked a lot of questions which I answered, and which filled a whole notebook. We decided to put the notes into a 40-day course.

And so the book you now hold in your hands? Well, here it is.

Lisa shares the direct healing experiences she had with the exercises contained in the 40-days of this book. She wrote 40 blog articles based on conversations we had with each other. These articles reveal a simple way out of food addiction. She also shares the beauty, principles and practical ideas of *A Course in Miracles.*

This is really the source of my realization and subsequent healing: ***that I cannot be anything else than blessed and free in my Innocence.***

This information is the book.

I am so grateful for you showing up in my life, that you may receive your healing, as well... that you may recognize your Innocence, Beauty, and inner Joy.

It is all I ever wanted. I feel continuous healing from this 40-day course and I am with you in it. I would like this 40-day book to be the support for you that you always wanted, and it is my desire as well to be available for you when you need more guidance, or just a place to laugh or cry or to be you.

For I know you as the amazing Light that you are. And I would like to celebrate it with you always.

Thanks for the invitation to be with you for a moment.

I love you.

Marielle School

Are you ready to be healed of food addiction?

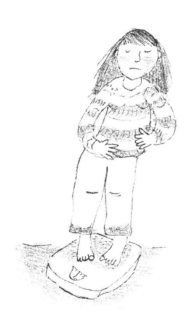

It Matters Totally is a 40-Day Program to heal food addiction with *a Course in Miracles.*

This program has nothing to do with food. There's no diet. You can throw away your scale (or at least put it in the closet!)

It Matters Totally is a program that supports you as you take little steps toward self-care and joy.

It is a program to help you come to know yourself as precious, lovable and valuable. It will give you the courage to say to yourself: "Hi, my friend, I'm so glad you are here." And to see what happens out of that.

It might be the first time in your life that you are willing to nurture yourself and be kind to yourself. You will feel a spark of love when you take that simple action.

You'll be amazed by how easily fear, sabotage, procrastination and high expectations will dissolve to make way for joy and appreciation.

It Matters Totally provides the opportunity to make new friends and share your discoveries with others that join you in the same journey.

We cover 40 topics in 40 days.

We believe in this program whole-heartedly because we have seen that it works. If you have a real desire to be healed of food addiction, this book can help you.

Week One is about Nurturing – it is your first attempt to be your own best friend. It is about learning to support yourself, to honor your sensitivity and to see the dramatic changes that arise from feelings of gratitude.

Week Two is about Self-Acceptance, something that has probably been absent from your life for a very long time. Now you can play with it and enjoy YOU and have fun.

Week Three is a dedication to Communication. It is about learning to relax and feel connected and loved.

Week Four is focused on Creativity - to find your own expression and to begin experimenting with it. To ask yourself the question: "What do I like??"

Week Five is about Receiving. To receive the grace of life and to feel the natural flow of it. To be open to receive all the gifts that are in store for you!

Week Six is a tribute to Joy. It is about allowing yourself to laugh and to say to yourself (and really mean it!): "It's okay, you can be happy now. You deserve it."

It is a privilege for us to be able to offer this program.

This is not a diet. Rather, it is a program for healing and happiness.

Are you ready?

PREPARATION: 40 Days of Passion & Purpose

Healing Food Addiction with *A Course in Miracles*

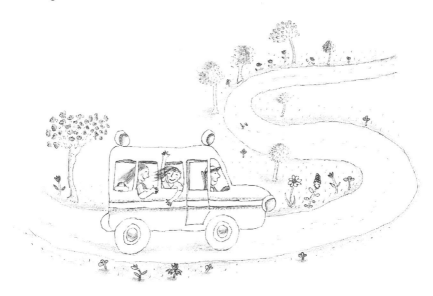

Marielle and I decided on 40 Days and 40 Topics because of Jesus' experience in the desert. He went into a space where he was able to LET GO OF THE PAST and LET GO OF THE FUTURE. From what I've read, Jesus had no idea how long he would be in the desert. He had no idea what would happen there. He didn't plan to go for "40 days" - he just went knowing that when he emerged he would be completely different.

The "desert experience" could have lasted a day or it could have lasted his whole lifetime. Jesus had NO IDEA going in WHAT TO EXPECT. But he knew he had come to a crossroads in his life where he had to make a CLEAN-BREAK from all that had come before.

Welcome to *It Matters Totally*. We want you to enter one way, having no expectations about what will occur, yet knowing you will emerge completely different.

We love the idea of a clean slate and a fresh new beginning. But where in this life - in this crazy hectic fast-paced life - does one have an opportunity to BREAK TIES WITH THE PAST and BREAK TIES WITH THE FUTURE?

That is the idea of this 40-Day Program. Within these "40 days", you set up an arbitrary space where you have the freedom to say "Okay, enough is enough. I'm ready to let go of conflict and self-hatred." And then you are hopefully able to communicate to your family and friends that you're going on a 40-Day Retreat (without leaving home) and that "things are going to be a little different from now on."

This 40-Day Program is about finding your true authentic self. It's about giving yourself the gift of freedom from all your routines and old ideas. It is a time "to draw your circle" as Jesus did in the desert, and for healing to occur.

Now, we understand it might not always work out ideally that way. Everyone has jobs and families and routines. We know it is impossible to create a real "desert experience" with an online program and a book. But we also know that IN GOD ALL THINGS ARE POSSIBLE.

It is our belief that it is not necessary to go to the mountaintop or into isolation to find peace and freedom. We believe each and everyone has the power to push a RE-START BUTTON in their life - right in the thick of it - and begin IN THAT VERY MOMENT with A BRAND NEW BEGINNING.

We offer to you that it is possible to come squarely into this day, and say: "I HAVE NO IDEA WHAT MY HABITS OR ROUTINES ARE ANYMORE. I AM GOING TO ALLOW EVERYTHING TO BE REVEALED TO ME NOW."

And that's a beautiful thing.

This program is about awareness. It is about finding passion and purpose in every single day, starting right from Day 1, and beginning to take care of yourself, nurture yourself, and do things that fill you with joy and happiness. In awareness, you begin to notice habits and routines that don't serve you - things you're doing on auto-pilot, unconsciously. The miracle occurs in letting those self-defeating habits go.

The miracle is that you are CHANGED IN THE TWINKLING OF AN EYE ... BORN AGAIN ... BRAND NEW.

Marielle and I have both been healed of food addiction because of this 40-Day Program. The addiction to overeat, diet and loathe ourselves has been healed completely.

So this 40-Day Program is about hitting the RE-START button in your life. It is about creating a clean space for yourself to allow something new to emerge.

This is your 40-Days.

It is your adventure into a CLEAN NEW SPACE; A NEW BEGINNING. And whenever you allow yourself to receive a gift like that, something really surprising and miraculous comes out of it.

This journey is about EXTREME SELF-CARE. You deserve the best. Because of this 40-Day Program I no longer cling to scraps of fear anymore. I remain always in the decision to love myself and to be happy and nice to myself. The food addiction is gone, and I no longer experience all the conflict I had experienced for so many years.

It's a new beginning. Each moment is a treasure. The "healing" that occurs is contained in becoming consciously aware of what a gift your life really is.

xoxoxoxoxoxoxo

In preparation we ask only one thing before you begin your 40 days: buy a paper journal for yourself. The main aspect of It Matters Totally is Extreme Self-Care. We ask you to begin to find ways to nurture yourself, to love yourself, and be nice to yourself. To a food addict that can sound like an impossible undertaking!! We know!! So, our first exercise guides you in taking one little baby step in the direction of your healing; it is a request that you do something really nice for yourself! We ask you to buy yourself a really beautiful journal, something gorgeous that makes your heart sing. This is your first gift to yourself. This signifies your willingness to be committed to your own healing.

This 40-day program is about your transformation.

Remember: This is an inward journey.

This 40-Day Program is a sacred space for you to begin having a loving relationship with yourself and to learn how to become your own best friend.

We ask simply that you follow the instructions for the daily topic and write in your paper journal every day. It's a simple program. And it works. You will be healed of food addiction if you make a solid commitment to yourself. All you need is "a little willingness" to let go of old ideas of hatred and see things in a brand new light.

A paper journal will help you start creating a nurturing friendship with yourself. Just you, with you. Pen and paper and you. Then to see what comes out of that.

You'll be amazed.

With all my love,

Lisa

WEEK 1
NURTURING

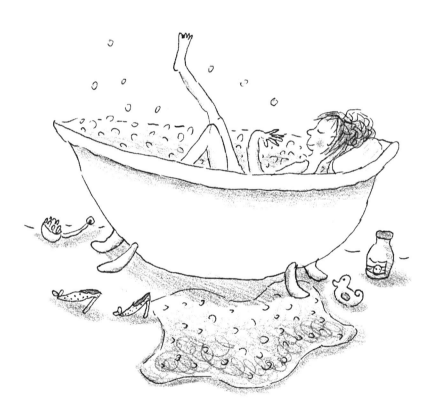

Day 1

Commitment

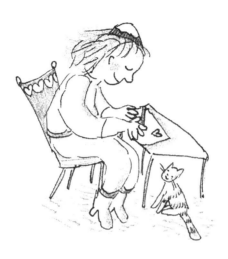

Today is your first day.

Welcome!!

This first step is always the most difficult and the scariest, but you have taken it now, and you are on your way! Congratulations! You have taken the most important step towards your own healing.

Thank you for taking this leap of faith into the unknown.

Today is about Commitment.

It is about your commitment to spend 40 days remembering your perfection. It is your commitment to remember the truth that God created you as His precious child.

You are whole, healed, perfect, wonderful, brilliant and magnificent.

Jesus says you are the light of the world. Do you think he is lying? Or is this statement true?

YOU ARE THE LIGHT OF THE WORLD.

We know you've tried other programs, diets, workshops, and have made other attempts to solve your problem. Perhaps you've gone through *A Course in Miracles,* through all 365 lessons, and gave it your best shot.

We know you have spent a lot of money trying to find a solution to your problem or addiction. We know you've talked to people, therapists, and groups about how to be happy and successful. We know you've bought books. We know you've listened to tapes.

You've searched and searched and searched.

We know! We did exactly the same thing. We searched and searched for a solution that worked. We know about those resolutions and promises. We also know about the frustration and pain of failure.

We know you've tried 1000 things 1000 ways and in the end... nothing really worked. Be honest. Did any of your attempts really work? Most likely you found yourself back where you started before you began, or maybe even a little bit worse off.

We know.

But there is one other thing we know – that at a certain stage you can't escape from your purpose. You've been called by God to remember your Identity as Light, Love, Joy and Happiness.

You made a promise before time even began to be that precious, brilliant child of Light that God created. It's a memory that has been buried for a long time, and yet there is something in you that KNOWS; something that keeps pushing you forward to change, to remember.

You know, with every cell in your body, that something is fundamentally wrong with your condition here in time and space. You know! I know! Everyone knows! There is something wrong with this world.

And so you keep trying to change. You change your address. You change your diet. You attempt to change your behavior. You change your relationships. You change your job. You're trying to get somewhere. You keep trying to make something happen.

And nothing changes!

Isn't this interesting???? No matter how much you try to change yourself, you're always the same.

And so at a certain point, you are likely to give up. It's exhausting to keep trying and failing.

So, this time around, here in the next 40 days, we're going to ask that you simply relax. RELAX LIKE YOU ARE ON A HOLIDAY.

Forget your plans. Forget your diets. Forget your attempts to quit sugar. Forget all attempts to change your behavior. Forget what you think the outcome is supposed to look like. You are free now.

Be free.

Little kids don't monitor their behavior and neither should you.

Today, on Day 1, we're going to ask you to do something really simple: make a commitment to the 40 days to be a little precious child of God. We ask you to make a commitment to take care of yourself, and to allow other people to take care of you

Make a commitment.

Exercise #1:

Write yourself a letter about your commitment.

Take out a piece of paper or really beautiful stationery and write a letter to yourself. You can type it on a typewriter, the computer, or you can handwrite it on stationery or notebook paper. Do whatever feels most comfortable to you.

This is your letter of commitment to yourself. Use your own words. You can write it as a love letter, a contract, an agreement, a reminder, or a few simple words. This is your own private letter and you should write it in a way that feels good to you.

Your letter is for those moments when you are halfway through the 40 days (or on Day 2!) when you start to forget why you dedicated yourself to this!

Lesson 28 from *A Course in Miracles* is entitled: "Above all else I want to see things differently."

The lesson begins: "Today we are really giving specific application to the idea for yesterday. [Above all else I want to see.] In these practice periods, you will be making a series of DEFINITE COMMITMENTS. The question of whether you will keep them in the future is NOT OUR CONCERN HERE. If you are willing at least to make them now, you have started on the way to keeping them. And we are still at the beginning."

> *If you are willing at least to make these commitments now, you have started on the way to keeping them. And we are still at the beginning.*

Day 2

Dedication to your Spirit

Have you bought yourself the perfect journal? Have you written your commitment letter to yourself?

Perhaps you're feeling a little overwhelmed.

This program is intense (we know!) but it works if you take some time to do the little that is asked. You'll see dramatic results that will take your breath away.

Today's exercise is to read your commitment letter out loud to yourself, preferably in front of the mirror. Hear the words that come from your heart, from the deepest part of yourself. Yesterday you wrote your commitment down on paper and today you are going to read it out loud and let yourself HEAR the importance of your words, in your own voice.

Often in addiction, we don't take ourselves too seriously. We think we don't have a voice. We think we're not heard. We think no one cares. We think that other people have all the opportunities and talent and they deserve abundance, happiness and recognition, but not us! We think that what we say doesn't matter very much.

Also, we addicts often don't MAKE time for ourselves as Spirit. When was the last time you took an hour every day (or even two or three!) just for fun and relaxation? If you don't take time for yourself every single day to remember and honor your playful creative Spirit, you will end up feeling overwhelmed, irritable, cranky and tired.

But *IT MATTERS TOTALLY.*

You matter totally.

What you do matters totally.

Your life matters totally.

What you say matters totally.

You make a difference in the world.

Today, you are going to begin honoring and paying attention to that innermost part of you that *is* you: Spirit.

All addictions are really a dedication to the body. Now we are going to shift that dedication from body-identification to Spirit-Identification.

It's not the food that's making you sick (or overweight, tired, or depressed), it's guilt and dedication to the body.

"The glitter of guilt you laid upon the body would KILL it. For what the ego loves, it kills for its obedience. But what obeys it not, it CANNOT kill. You have ANOTHER dedication which would keep the body incorruptible and perfect as long as it is useful for your holy purpose."
Urtext, Chapter 19, The Incorruptible Body

Do you see that? You have ANOTHER dedication that would keep the body incorruptible and perfect as long as it is useful for your holy purpose.

An incorruptible, perfect body! Amazing, right? It is your inheritance to have a perfect incorruptible body as long as the body is used for the Holy Spirit's holy purpose.

It also says: "PARTIAL DEDICATION IS IMPOSSIBLE."

So the exercise for today is about being dedicated to your Spirit. Up until now you've been dedicated to your body. But now we are asking you to take the focus off the body and be dedicated to Spirit.

It's not necessary for you to find out what your holy purpose is. It's only necessary that you make another dedication... a dedication to your Spirit.

Say to yourself:

"I will accept my part in God's plan for salvation. We dedicate ourselves to truth today."
ACIM, Lesson 98, I will accept my part in God's plan
for salvation.

WE DEDICATE OURSELVES TO TRUTH TODAY.

"If you find resistance strong and dedication weak, you are not ready. DO NOT FIGHT YOURSELF. But think about the kind of day you want and tell yourself that there is a way by which this very day can happen just like that."
Urtext, Chapter 30, Rules for Decision Making

THINK ABOUT THE KIND OF DAY YOU WANT.

THINK ABOUT THE KIND OF SPACE YOU WANT.

THINK ABOUT THE KIND OF LIFE YOU WANT.

And then tell yourself that there is a way by which this very day (space, life) can happen just like that.

You can also use your journal to write about these things you want. Have fun!

Exercise #1:

Read your commitment letter out loud.

Exercise #2

Create a space for yourself.

This place should be comfortable, inviting, beautiful, quiet and peaceful. This exercise is NOT about getting rid of clutter. It's NOT about fixing what is broken. It's NOT about changing aspects of yourself (or your life) that are unacceptable. This exercise is about CREATION. All too often, addicts don't really take care of themselves. They accept the scraps and crumbs. They give and they give and they give, always taking second-best in order to help other people. Most addicts take the smaller piece, the smaller space, in order to appear not too greedy or too selfish. They try to appear like they don't have any needs or wants. And most addicts give such a good performance convincing other people that they have no needs that eventually they convince even themselves that they don't need much!

Eventually, they (we) start believing that whatever comes our way is acceptable and good, even if it's an already chewed-up, half-eaten bone!

You take the crappy apartment. You settle for second-best. You live in less-than-perfect conditions. You struggle and try to make yourself fit into one little corner of life. All the while you're quietly saying to yourself "It's okay. I'm fine. I'm good. I don't need anything."

Well YOU might not need anything, but your Spirit wants everything. Today is about being dedicated to your Spirit.

Your Spirit wants to be heard, honored and recognized. It's time to start paying attention to that small, still voice in you that longs to be heard. It's time to start accepting your inheritance which was given to you by God in your creation.

Jesus in *A Course in Miracles* says, "You do not ask too much of life, but far too little."
    ACIM, Lesson 133, I will not value what is valueless.

"Ask for EVERYTHING of the Holy Spirit, because YOUR requests to Him are real, being of your right mind. Would the Holy Spirit deny the Will of God?"
    Urtext, Chapter 9, The Acceptance of Reality

You're going to take the focus off how you can help other people, and you are going to start paying attention to your Spirit... to you! This is your time!

So today, you are going to give yourself the gift of a great space, a space that is all your own. This space is your OASIS, your ISLAND, your PARADISE, a place that is uniquely yours.

Be creative. Put things you love in this space.

What do you love? For me it includes photos of friends and family, pictures of my dogs and cats, a coffee table with my favorite books, lots of pillows, a glass vase that contains beautiful white rocks that I picked up on a beach in Greece, a framed photo of a Calvin & Hobbes cartoon that makes me laugh like crazy every time I see it, a box of treasured love letters, a comfy blanket, a bowl of chocolate, and gorgeous fresh flowers that I buy at the Farmer's Market every Thursday for $5. These are a few of my favorite things.

Most addicts have no idea what they like or dislike. Their entire focus for their entire life has been about pleasing others and holding up an appearance. They never took the time to find out what *they* liked. This lesson is all about you. What do you love?

Also, we ask you to put a childhood photo of you in this space. That child is you!

That brilliant, fabulous child is you!

Day 3

Finding your own space
instead of isolating

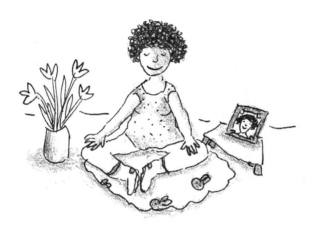

Today is a continuation of yesterday's exercise to set up your own space.

I think it is safe to say that most addicts are easily overwhelmed. It's a little bit like being schizophrenic – you are ONE WAY when you are with people or in crowds or social settings, and you're ANOTHER WAY when you are alone by yourself.

And that's because you never had space.

The addict is always hiding, constantly searching for ways to become invisible and minimize needs while secretly longing to be heard, seen, loved and appreciated.

The addict puts other people first and then takes what is left over.

This kind of behavior is intolerable to the Spirit.

The only way the addict knows how to cope and replenish is by isolating. They can't wait to get away from people to be alone so that they can relax and be themselves.

It's a bit like the actor on stage that spends all his energy giving the performance of his lifetime, and the second he is offstage, he heaves a sigh of relief. He can let down his guard because the audience can't see him anymore. He's free to be himself. He takes off the costume and makeup because there is no one around to judge him, no one to please and to perform for.

Sound familiar??

So today we are going to encourage you to start becoming comfortable with your body, as you are now, and to bridge the gap between the way you are when you are alone versus the way you are when you are with people.

And the first exercise towards bridging this gap is to find your own space instead of isolating; to find that place of calm within the storm.

Today's first exercise is: MASSAGE and BREATHING.

What is the purpose of this exercise? To begin to get to know yourself as you are today.

The addict is always waiting for a future moment to like himself. He's always disconnected from the present moment. The mind is always on the next intriguing encounter, the piece of cake he'll let himself have when he's home alone, the next diet that will transform his life.

Always thinking about something "in the future"; never being here now.

SPACE.

Today's lesson is about space. You think if you were in a different space things would be better, different, improved, happier, more peaceful.

A Course in Miracles says you are "constantly striving, never arriving."

Constantly striving, never arriving. Sounds familiar???

So today, right now, we ask that you start becoming comfortable with your body and comfortable with your space.

Exercise #1

Connect with your body through massage and breathing:

> Please take a breath. Breathe. Big deep breath.
> Breathe in. Breathe out. Gentle. Relax.
>
> Again. Breathe. You're good enough now. You're
> perfect as you are now. Breathe.

Now, take your hands and feel every part of your body. Massage your hands, your arms, your legs, your feet. Connect with your body. Stand up. Stretch. Breathe. Place your hand over your heart and feel your heartbeat. Feel your breath. Become aware of the wonder and the beauty that is your body. No matter how much you hate it, it's working perfectly! All the cells are continually rejuvenating themselves. Blood is coursing through your veins. Food breaks down into fuel and energy. And you don't have to do anything to make this happen!!

You're able to walk and talk and move and stretch, and get from one room to the other room with relative ease.

You say you hate your body, but it's a perfect instrument! It's a miracle!

Exercise #2

BECOME AWARE OF YOUR LANGUAGE AND USE OF WORDS.

Look at what kinds of statements you say a lot. Many addicts spend half the day saying "I'm sorry." They carry a lot of guilt around just for taking up space, or speaking out loud.

"I'm fine." "I'm okay." "I'm good." "I don't need help." I'm sorry."

Addicts crave love, appreciation and recognition.

They think the only way to get this love and appreciation is to be "good" and to "give, give, give, give, give."

They give in order to get. They think if they give enough eventually someone will return the love they crave.

Addiction is a craving. You think you crave food or a great body, but really what you are craving is love, appreciation and recognition.

So addicts put on a happy face. They say "I'm sorry" a lot. They try to be quiet and good. They "over-give", hoping to get.

But this is exhausting!!

Admit it. It's exhausting pretending you are okay when you are not. It's tiring trying to constantly take care of other people when really you just wish someone would take care of you!

So today, you're starting to get to know yourself.

You're starting to take care of yourself and to allow yourself to be taken care of by others, by the simple recognition that you are loved and lovable and that you deserve it.

A Course in Miracles says: "God longs to give you everything."

You never really had an opportunity to allow God to give to you because you were so busy filling the space, trying to please other people with your giving. You've never really left open a clean empty space to receive.

That's right, receiving. The #1 most difficult thing for an addict to do!

This 40-day program is about coming to know yourself as God created you.

Exercise #3

Find out what kind of person you are in your own space. How do you move in this space, knowing that it is all your own?

Did you set up a space for yourself? How does it feel? What do you feel?

Day 4

Trusting/being yourself

Today's lesson is about trust and being yourself.

Most addicts have no idea who they are. They've been so busy/preoccupied trying to please other people that they are nothing more than a blurred image of what they think they are supposed to be: good, kind, quiet, happy, responsible and helpful.

Duh. Boring!!!!!!

The addict is a great liar. He spends almost his entire life lying. Lies, Lies, Lies. No wonder you overeat, smoke, drink, sedate and sabotage yourself.

No wonder you're in pain. You've been denying yourself your entire life!

Your Spirit knows you're lying, knows you're being inauthentic. You've not been true to yourself and you've never really given yourself a fair chance.

For example:

- You do things that you don't want to do.
- You say "yes" when really you mean "no."
- You overexert yourself.
- You act like you have lots of energy when really you would like to take a nap or relax and have someone else take care of you.
- You smile and act holy when you feel like tearing someone's head off.

- You send contradictory messages. You say "I'm okay" when you are not okay. You say "I don't need help" when you do. You say "I'm fine" when you're not fine.

This is lying.

As I pointed out yesterday, this kind of behavior is intolerable to the Spirit. It's intolerable to You.

Today's lesson is about trust and being yourself.

Trust enough to be vulnerable, to be exposed, and to be yourself. It's about coming clean with yourself, and being honest.

Trust is the first characteristic of a Teacher of God.
Honesty is the second characteristic.
Tolerance is the third.
Gentleness is the fourth.
Joy is the fifth.
Defenselessness is the sixth.
Generosity is the seventh.
Patience is the eighth.
Faithfulness is the ninth.
Open-Mindedness is the tenth.

Trust, Honesty, Patience, Gentleness. Keep it simple.

The addict is full of fear. The addict is afraid of exposure, afraid of making a mistake.

Most addicts are total perfectionists. It's exhausting to hold up an image of yourself and never let down your guard.

Trust.

Trust that you can begin to know yourself as God created you: pure light.

You don't ever have to explain yourself to anyone. You are perfectly free to be yourself. You're free to make mistakes. You're free to let yourself get messy.

Kids let themselves get messy and so should you. Don't worry about mud or spilled milk; it washes off. If you want to put your hands and feet in paint, go right ahead.

Exercise #1:

Today we want you to think of something you have always wanted but denied yourself. Today, we want you to make this thing/experience yours. It could be something you have wanted to buy but have put off because you have been taking care of debts or other people. It could be something you really wanted as a child but never received. It could be a characteristic that you've always wanted but which you thought you didn't deserve.

Today, do this thing you have always wanted to do. At a minimum, start thinking about what you want and make a decision that you are going to get it for yourself.

Last week I received birthday money and I bought a bicycle! It is a miracle for me to spend money on myself. For the past 20 years, I have been a "responsible adult", paying debts and bills when money comes my way.

But last week I bought a bicycle!

I let the kid in me have what she really, really wanted for her birthday! I also bought a Barbie! When was the last time you were in the toy aisle???

When was the last time you were in an art store?
When was the last time you were in a candy store?
When was the last time you were in a bookstore?

When was the last time you took the kid in you out to play?

I love Carlos Castaneda. He talks about "the art of stalking." Stalking is where you figure out what you want and stalk it. You learn what your bad habits are, and you stalk them. You hunt them down, stalk them, and kill them. You learn about the way your mind works. You start to become aware of the areas where you trip up (fight with the spouse always leads you to eat a bag of cookies). You begin learning about yourself. You begin learning your likes and dislikes. Hunters stalk animals. A good hunter learns the habits of the animal he is stalking. He's always one step ahead. Warriors stalk themselves. They learn everything they can about themselves. In order to be a good stalker, you need to know what you want and how you're going to get it.

A true hunter discards all unnecessary acts. He knows what he wants. He knows what he doesn't want. He's certain and calm. He goes after what he wants (and avoids what he doesn't want) and he achieves success. Plain and simple.

Exercise #2:

Begin stalking the characteristics that you want for yourself. Most people with food addiction have an image of how they want to be when they are their perfect weight. They feel they'll be more courageous, more adorable, wear nicer clothes, be more authentic, and have more energy to do fun things. They'll go hiking, swimming, be beautiful and creative. They'll be the kind of person who goes to fabulous restaurants. They'll take care of themselves better.

Today's exercise is to become these characteristics today. You're it already!

All the things you want "in the future" are available to you today.

The addict is result-oriented, always focusing on that far-away future-date when life is perfect. Always striving, never arriving.

Now we are asking you to: FOCUS ON YOUR THOUGHTS. FOCUS ON FEELING GOOD.

It's not about doing it right anymore.

Be willing to make mistakes.

Be willing to look like a fool.

Be willing to trust your own impulses.

Be willing to listen to what you really want.

Be willing to let go of images of how you are supposed to be.

WHAT DOES THE LITTLE CHILD IN YOU NEED?
WHAT IS THIS CHILD LIKE?
WHAT DOES THIS CHILD WANT?

How do you feel?

Day 5

Honoring your sensitivity

Most addicts are super sensitive.

They are easily overwhelmed, get tired easily, need lots of time alone for resting and relaxing, have low tolerance for malls, parties, social settings, groups of people, and loud noise.

The reason for this is sensitivity.

You're sensitive to energies. *This is good!*

It means you are connected with Spirit. It means you are operating beyond the five senses of touch, taste, sound, sight, and smell.

To be sensitive is to be able to feel energy.

But somewhere along the way you learned that being sensitive was wrong, bad, shameful. In order to cope, you learned to operate on two speeds: High and Low.

You learned how to behave with people. You learned how to "get along" in order to be liked. You learned how to be charming, nice, good, friendly and to hold an intelligent conversation so that people didn't think you were weird or rude.

And what was the result? Exhaustion. Not honoring your Self. Not listening to your basic needs. Ignoring the small, still voice that tells you to go find a quiet place and relax.

In other words: You've been trying to be someone that you are not. It's hard work keeping up an appearance!

For most addicts, there is no middle ground. There's no balance. Either you are ON or you are OFF.

You've either got tons of energy or no energy – there's no in-between.

You probably are intuitive, psychic, or have artistic abilities that you've been ignoring most of your life.

So today on Day 5, the topic is: HONORING YOUR SENSITIVITY.

The difficulty most addicts have is that they are ashamed of their sensitivity. They think it's wrong. They try to act normal in groups of people when they'd rather be home alone. They tolerate loud music even though it's making them cringe inside.

They try and try and try and try to be like other people (who seemingly have no problem in groups, parties, and interacting with people) but it never really works. You'd rather be home alone with a drink, a cigarette or a bag of chips.

Today we are asking you to become aware of your energy levels. We're not asking you to fix anything. We're not asking you to change.

Today, starting now, we'd like to ask you to start HONORING YOUR SENSITIVITY.

It's a gift to be sensitive. You're not like other people. So stop trying to fit in. You don't fit in. You'll never fit in.

And that's your gift!

To be sensitive means to be tuned into Spirit.

Most addicts are exceptionally gifted and creative. They are the musicians, artists, and writers.

But look what they do to themselves! They drink, smoke, kill themselves, cut off their ears, and stick their heads in gas ovens. They are unable to pace themselves. They are unable to find a balance between living in the world and entering into the realm of creation.

You probably feel like an alien: misunderstood, lost, cold, and far away from home.

You *are* an alien. YOU'RE NOT LIKE OTHER PEOPLE. This is good!

Today's exercises are about:

> -honoring your boundaries
> -becoming aware of your energy levels
> -protecting your energy/sensitivity by honoring it
> -pacing yourself
> -saying no
> -not explaining yourself

These exercises take courage and discipline.

The addict tries to do everything. He/She tries to be the perfect husband, wife, mother, daughter, son, father. The addict is mostly a loner, but attempts to "be normal" by acting in ways that are "socially acceptable."

You can stop pretending now. This world is not your home. You don't belong here. Now you can begin honoring your sensitivity. Celebrate it, cherish it!

You are Spirit!

Exercise #1:

Watch your energy levels. Become aware of your highs and lows. Start noticing when you are being drained. How long can you hold a conversation before you start getting tired? How long can you stay at a party? How long can you tolerate loud noise?

<u>Exercise #2:</u>

Say "no" when you mean "no."

Practice saying "no" when you don't want to do something. If you don't want to do something, stop saying "yes" to it.

"No" is really easy to say with some practice.

"No, I'm not interested."
"No, I'm busy."
"No, I'm tired."
"No."
"Thanks, but no thanks."
"No."

The tremendous healing power of "NO"! You don't have to explain yourself. "No" is sufficient.

Most addicts say "yes" when really they mean "no."

You are a gifted, talented, creative child of God. You have gifts that are buried, lying dormant, just waiting for you to discover them.

And you will never discover your gifts while you waste your energy trying to please other people.

It's great to spend time being alone and honoring your sensitivity. You're an artist!

Artists don't need to explain themselves. Artists need space and quiet to tap into their own God-given talents.

You're brilliant.

This is the new you.

Now, instead of trying to fit in with other people's ideas of what you should be, we ask you to:

- listen to yourself
- pay attention to your energy levels and get a sense of your own natural energy rhythm
- don't waste your time pleasing people (if people think you are rude because you said "NO!" and didn't explain yourself ... Good!)
- honor your sensitivity

Celebrate your sensitivity!

Exercise #3:

In your journal, write about what you really want to do once you're able to create more time for yourself.

What would your day be like if you weren't so busy taking care of other people?

Write about situations you don't want to handle. Write about things you don't want to do.

Day 6

Nourishment

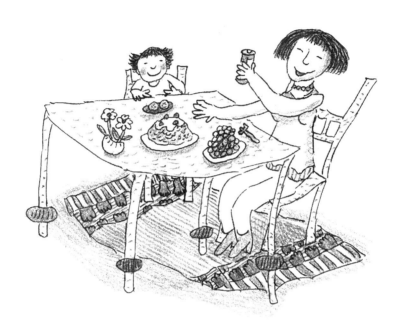

Today's lesson is about NOURISHMENT.

It is about meeting basic needs.
It is about warmth.
It is about surrounding yourself with supportive people that respect and encourage you.

It's time to start taking care of yourself the way you would take care of a newborn baby.

We want you to think about this. Would you starve a newborn baby? Would you force feed this child? How would you care for it?

Mostly, you would watch for signals. A child knows what it needs. It doesn't come up with plans or diets. It knows what it needs.

When a child is hungry, it cries as loudly as possible.
When a child is tired, it becomes cranky.

And yet many adults ignore the natural impulses of their body.

I go hours and hours without eating and then I'm starving and I reach for the fastest thing I can find: a bowl of cereal, french fries, a candy bar. Would I feed a child this way?

No, I would not, and yet it's the way I feed myself. Then I'm surprised when my body is not working at optimal levels. All the signs are there of a vehicle operating on gas fumes: I'm tired. I have low energy. I'm bitchy. My lips are cracked and dry. I'm bloated. My skin is discolored.

Warning signals that something needs to shift.

What is a good practical thing to do for this child that needs to eat more regularly than I have been feeding her? I can start checking in more regularly, become more aware, and start carrying food with me – the way a mother always carries food for her children.

There are simple, practical things I can do to start taking better care of myself.

Is your body sending you signals? Are you sick? Is your body failing you?

Then it's time to start nourishing yourself. It's time to start taking care of yourself.

It's time to stop controlling and manipulating your emotions and all the while saying, "I'm okay."
What nourishes you?

This question is not just about food. What nourishes you? It could be sitting out in the sun, reading a book, taking a yoga class, playing with a pet, going to a cafe with a friend, taking a bubble bath.

Most addicts do not take care of themselves properly. They are not connected to their body. Most addicts have no respect for their bodies. They feel only self-hatred and rejection, wishing and waiting for some future time when they will like themselves.

Waiting for a moment which never arrives!

They are starving themselves of the love that would heal them. You've been starving yourself.

What you need is love, support, appreciation and respect.

I read an article saying that people who are overweight are malnourished. I thought that was interesting. I always thought it was children in Africa who were malnourished, emaciated and starving. But really, it was me!

I was starving myself... while I was stuffing myself!

So today, start thinking of ways to nourish yourself.
What nourishes you? What would it mean to take care of yourself?

Exercise #1:

Start nourishing that newborn baby that is you.

A Course in Miracles says you are REBORN IN CHRIST and that YOU ARE A TINY NEWCOMER. And this Christ child in you *needs* your loving care.

"You are a Child of God, a priceless part of His Kingdom, which He created as part of Him. Nothing else exists, and ONLY this is real."
Urtext, Chapter 6, The Only Answer

We ask you to find a warm, soft cuddly blanket for the newborn child in you. This child is in your care and is your responsibility. Yes, you are now officially a mother or a father. Congratulations! You have a beautiful child to take care of. That child lives in you! That child, as well, *is* you!

Welcome to the world, little one!

Jesus, in *A Course in Miracles,* says to you: "Child of God, you were created to create the good, the beautiful, and the holy."
Urtext, Chapter 1, Distortions of Miracle Impulses

"Holy Child of God, when will you learn that ONLY holiness can content you, and give you peace?"
Urtext, Chapter 15, Be Not Content with Littleness

Yes, this little child is dependent on your holy relationship – with yourself, and then as well, with your brothers in Christ. This child is dependent upon your holiness, upon you loving yourself.

Now that you have a newborn child to take care of, you need some additional support. Nobody should have to take care of a baby alone. Depend then, on your holy relationships!

Exercise #2:

Start putting together a support team. Think of people who support, love, respect and encourage you. This is your team – an absolute essential part of healing.

Exercise #3:

Write down three things that nourish you and do them today.

Day 7

Gratitude

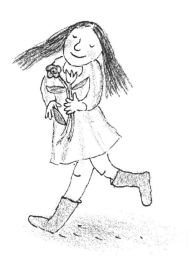

Today's lesson is about Gratitude.

Most addicts (heck, most people!) focus on what is wrong, rather than focusing on what is right.

They focus on:

> -the problem rather than the solution
> -the negative rather than on the positive
> -grievances instead of gratitude
> -what is wrong rather than what is right
> -what is lacking/missing

It takes a CONSCIOUS DECISION to shift your focus.

It's like turning the dial on the radio station. You were on one station that was getting a lot of static and poor reception and now we are asking you to turn that dial to a frequency of love and gratitude.

Today, we want you to write a love letter to yourself. Make it the most incredible love letter that has ever been sent in the history of the world.

Write down everything you like about yourself.

Write down everything that you LOVE about yourself.

Write down how grateful you are to have yourself in your life, how lucky you are to know you, and then list all the reasons why you are so great, lovable, charming, beautiful, talented, sweet, funny, smart.

Write down everything you like/love about yourself.

Most addicts are so full of self-hatred and loathing that they cannot imagine they have even one good quality. Mostly they just hate themselves. They hate their life. They are bored, angry, full of doubt and completely disconnected from the truth of themselves.

PEOPLE WITH EATING DISORDERS HAVE NO IDEA WHAT IT IS LIKE TO HAVE A LIFE.

Addicts think everyone else is having all the fun. They are waiting for something big to occur. Only 9 times out of 10 they have no idea what they are waiting for!

The power of gratitude!

Gratitude will transform your life.

If you live in a horrible house, give thanks for it! Find everything that is great about it.

If you hate your body, find something that is awesome about it. It's a perfectly good working machine. Look at how miraculous your body really is! You say you hate it but it's a work of art! Look at what it is capable of!

You say you hate your thighs but look at what those legs are capable of! You say you hate your stomach all the while your heart is pumping, blood is flowing, cells are being renewed, toxins flushed out, and food is being digested. Yet all you can focus on is how you are too fat!

I laughed in amazement the first time I looked at this logically. My whole life my focus has been on the 30-50 pounds I would like to lose. That's all I've been focusing on!!! Talk about insanity.

I have the amazing ability to walk, talk, love, laugh, sing, write, see and hear. It amazes me that I can think a thought and then communicate it through my fingers on a keyboard! How wild is it to put thoughts on paper??? It's insane! It's huge! Most people take it for granted that you have eyes to see and ears to hear and the ability to think. These are gifts of the highest order! Everyone possesses these abilities.

And I'm thinking my butt is too big. LOL.

Everything gets put into perspective when you focus on gratitude.

I have a little technique I use when people are complaining about their problems. I say, "Tell me something good."

This disrupts their thinking. It throws everyone right off track. They were focusing on grievances and complaints and now I am asking them to switch the dial to gratitude.

Exercise #1:

Write yourself a love letter.

Exercise #2:

Stand in the spotlight today. Be a star. Stand in your own magnificence. Hold your head high. Realize how important you are. Recognize that you make a difference in the world. Stand in that grace and certainty.

Exercise #3:

Tell me something good.

WEEK 2

SELF
ACCEPTANCE

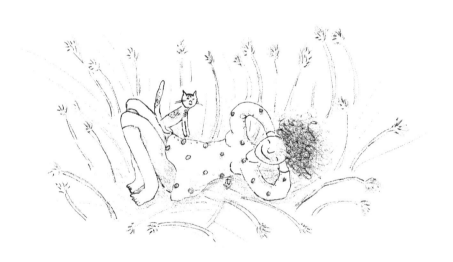

Day 8

Nature

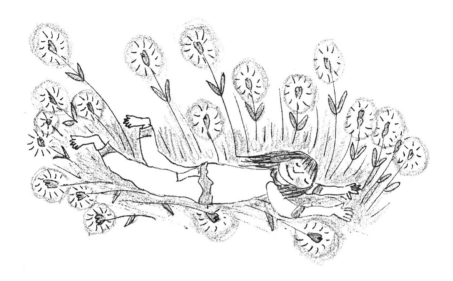

Most addicts feel isolated and disconnected.

They feel disconnected from their bodies. They feel disconnected from their life. They feel disconnected from other people.

And they attempt to connect! They try! They reach out. They help. They smile a lot. They listen. They give, give, give, give, GIVE! They are the most giving people on the planet. They are compassionate, gentle, kind and loving.

And yet... they still feel disconnected.

It's like something MAJOR-LEAGUE is missing.

So today's lesson, Day 8, is about NATURE, which is about CONNECTION.

Nature = Connection.

We are in Week 2 and the theme is Self-Acceptance. Being in nature is the beginning step to accepting your perfection.

The difficulty with trying to connect with people is that the experience is always fleeting. It's NOT consistent. You have one great moment of joy and connection with someone and then it's gone. They have other obligations. You have other obligations. You can't expect anyone to always be there for you 24 hours a day, 7 days a week, and to be gentle with you.

Well, guess what? NATURE WILL BE THERE FOR YOU 24 hours a day, 7 days a week. And she is always kind and generous. This is the reason it's great to start connecting with her. Nature is always there and she's entirely consistent. She's dependable! She's gorgeous! And she's right outside your door.

Today we're going to ask you to spend some time with her. But before we go to today's exercise, there's something I'd like to share with you.

We've been receiving letters and talking to individuals who have participated in this 40-day experience, and the #1 theme that has come up consistently is that people are too busy with other things to take time for themselves. Certain participants who determined to go the 40 days pulled back, ending up (seemingly) nowhere to be found! We've come to realize the seriousness of this disease. It is scary to think that you might be healed of food addiction! You've spent your whole life thinking about food, diets and weight. Who would you be without your addiction?

You cannot even begin to answer this question because you have no idea. It's like a void. It's like the loss of your personality. This can be terrifying! It's easier to stay busy and distracted than to do the work that will transform you.

The exercises of *It Matters Totally* can be the first baby steps to move you in a new direction.

Today, as we look at the idea of connecting with nature, let's look for a moment as well at some of the great things *A Course in Miracles* says about your relationship with her. Following are some incredible lines from Lesson 156, which is entitled "I walk with God in perfect holiness":

"There is a light in you which cannot die; whose presence is so holy that the world is sanctified by you. All things that live bring gifts to you, and offer them in gratitude and gladness at your feet. The scent of flowers is their gift to you. The waves bow down before you, and the trees extend their arms to shield you from the heat, and lay their leaves before you on the ground that you may walk in softness, while the wind sinks to a whisper round your holy head."

Nature loves you! The universe longs to behold you!

The lesson continues: "The light in you is what the universe longs to behold. All living things are still before you, for they recognize Who walks with them."

To stand in nature is to begin to know yourself as connected with something beautiful, magnificent, awesome and powerful.

To be in nature is to begin to experience a CONSISTENT CONNECTION.

Nature will never leave you. She loves you just the way you are. She rejoices that you came!

The wind embraces you.
The sun warms you.
The rain makes everything clean and new again.

Exercise #1:

GO OUTSIDE. Be in nature. Look around. See how perfect nature is even when she's messy! She's always herself!

Nature gives you back your place in creation. You are part of the totality of all that God created.

This is not a complicated lesson. We are not asking you to take a hike, and we're not asking you to go on a camping trip for the weekend. Just go outside.

Sit in the sun. Take off your shoes. Look at the flowers. Feel the wind. Take a walk to the mailbox. Walk around the yard. Walk around the block. Breathe. Look. Listen.

Notice how you feel in nature, and then ask yourself these questions:

- How *do* you feel?
- How does it feel to sit and relax and do nothing?
- Do you feel peaceful? Or do you feel agitated, as though you should be doing something?

Can you simply take a moment with nature today and just "be"?

Day 9

Freedom

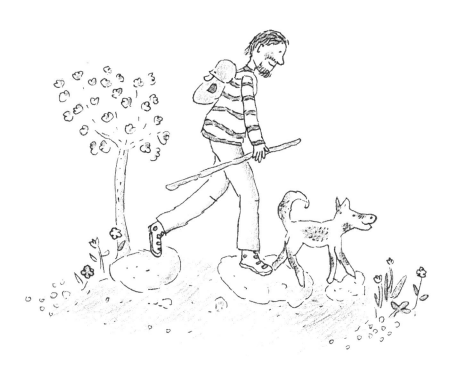

A Course in Miracles asks: "Do you want freedom of the body or of the mind? For both you cannot have."
  ACIM, Chapter 22, The Light of the Holy Relationship

Great question: Do you want freedom of the body or freedom of the mind? You can't have both.

Dedication to the body will keep you bound and limited; a prisoner. Most people do not realize they are a prisoner in their own life! They think they can only go certain places and do certain things. They think they are "not allowed" to ride a bicycle, or take a dance class, or go into certain stores or restaurants. They are not supposed to order dessert or eat from the bread basket, or wear certain types of clothes. They think they are supposed to act a certain way, keeping themselves in line at all times. Otherwise they will be punished (or worse, not liked!)

Um, excuse me... but welcome to the prison house!

You think you're supposed to get out of bed at a certain time, shower by a certain time, have your hair or makeup all in place. Then you shuffle in line for the routine to begin!

This is called "Prison."

You go through the motions of your day, behaving. You are a good little inmate. You behave and no one bothers you. You smile. You do as instructed. You follow the rules. You don't rock the boat.

You are a model prisoner. You get five stars!

But, be honest. Is this really what you want? Five stars for being the best prisoner?

The prison doors are open. You can walk out into the sunlight. You can have anything you want. You can do anything you want. You're free.

You're not a body. You're free.

To be truly free means that you are going to have to let go of the shackles and chains that are binding you.

Most prisoners (addicts) get used to a certain rhythm that they depend on. They may move very fast, always ahead of everyone else, always on their toes, one step ahead of the game. This type has a lot of nervous energy and likes to be productive and useful.

And then there is a second type of prisoner. This type moves very slowly. Having resigned and given up, this type is lethargic and not easily motivated and is often tired.

Both types have a rhythm.

A rhythm, according to the dictionary is "a movement or variation characterized by the regular recurrence of particular elements."

A rhythm follows a certain pattern. It is predictable.

Predictability is a defining characteristic of someone in prison. Their days follow an identical pattern, one to the next.

Are *you* predictable? Is your life a pattern?

Most addicts have a routine they stick with. Come hell or high water, you know what addicts are going to do! They play it safe. Their rhythm is comfortable and familiar, even while they are dying a slow and painful death due to boredom.

Exercise #1:

Ask yourself the following questions and answer them:

> -How free would you like your life to be?
> -What would your day look like?
> -What would you do in your ideal life?
> -How would you move?

Exercise #2:

Escape from the prison house.

Breaking free means movement! It means you are no longer going to sit around accepting "your fate" of a lifetime behind bars.

Choose one action/movement that is different from the way you normally do things, and begin it.

Do you go places just because you think it is expected? Then stop going. Do you wait for things to happen? Then start taking the steps to make things happen. Do you sit by the phone waiting for someone to call? Then pick up the phone and call him (or her) first. Do you sit inside all day waiting for an exciting adventure to occur? Then go outside and make your own fun. Do you always buy the same food week after week after week? Then buy something new. Go to a different store. Disrupt your routine. Disrupt your patterns. Disrupt your rhythm.

Movement. Get moving.

Time to break free. A prisoner who is escaping does not continue to sit in his prison cell. He moves! He plans! He plots! He has the tools he needs. He has the support he needs (because no prisoner can escape without inside help!) and he follows through.

So today, we ask you to disrupt your familiar energy patterns. Put on some music and dance. Move. Stretch. Breathe. Jump up and down. Do jumping jacks. Start moving that stagnant energy. Shake it out!

It also means you have to look at all the obstacles in your plan to making a clean get-away.

What obstacles are in your way to breaking free?

Day 10

Having your own voice

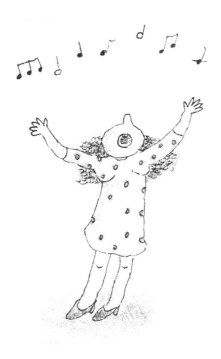

Your voice is all-powerful!

Do you realize that the sound of your voice creates a whole world? Everything is energy and the sound of your voice is an energy vibration.

What you say (the stories you tell, the way you talk about yourself, the way you talk about others) works like a magnet. If you speak negativity, negativity comes to you. If you speak from appreciation, beauty and love, you call these things to you.

Not many people realize this FACT. They falsely believe their words are neutral. They think they can say anything they want without any effect. Most people report on what their eyes and ears show them, and this kind of behavior is guaranteed to get you into a lot of trouble. The world you see and hear is illusion. Start to practice talking about truth instead of talking about illusion.

Do you realize you can filter your thoughts?
Do you realize you choose which thoughts become words out of your mouth?

You think it is innocent to say you are sick, fat, ugly, stupid. You think you are just reporting on the "facts." This is the most dangerous thing you can do! Be careful! Saying you hate yourself is more harmful than playing with fire and gasoline!

When you call yourself fat, ugly, sick or stupid, you are sending a signal to your cells. And your cells respond! Be careful.

Did you ever hear about the Dr. Emoto's experiment with water? (http://www.hado.net) He did an experiment where he took water samples from the same water source. He started talking to the different samples of water. He said "I love you" to one, "I hate you" to another, and "you make me sick" to yet another. In response to the intention or different emotion extended to each, various water crystals were formed.

Did you see this experiment? Mind-blowing.

Those that received vibrations of "you make me sick" turned brown and dead, and the crystals that received vibrations of "I love you" turned into beautiful formations.

If you can grasp the significance of THE POWER OF THE VIBRATION OF WORDS AND THE SOUND OF YOUR OWN VOICE, you will be able to transform your life. What you say affects you in every way!

When you were a child, did your mother or father ever wash your mouth out with soap?? I grew up in the 70s, a time when disciplining children was not yet known as child abuse. I was punished, sent to my room without dinner and had my mouth washed out with soap. I didn't like it, but one thing is for sure: I stopped talking filth.

Back when I was a kid, swear words and the word "hate" were off-limits. If I or my sisters said "hate", out came the soap!

I learned this little ditty when I was 4-years old:

> Don't say "hate"
> Your mother will faint
> Your father will fall into a bucket of paint
> Your sister will cry
> Your brother will die
> And all of your friends will say "goodbye!"

Pretty scary stuff to a 4-year old!! But I learned not to say the word "hate." It's not in my vocabulary.

Next time you call yourself "fat", "sick" or "unworthy", you should try washing your mouth out with soap. This is a great technique. Trust me, you won't like it. But it's very effective!

You can wash your mouth out with soap for gossiping, complaining, worrying and/or expressing negativity.

Become aware of your own voice. Become aware of the power of words.

Has it occurred to you that when you tell a story, you are the decision-maker of what details you tell?

To realize this is to claim back all your power!

Today's lesson is about finding your own voice, in truth.

Exercise #1:

Look at your use of language. Become aware of what comes out of your mouth. Awareness is always the first step. Most people have no idea they spend half their day complaining, worrying, and gossiping.

What is coming out of your mouth? Are you speaking the truth? Are you talking about God, love, appreciation, joy, and gratitude?

Or are you talking about time, space, sickness, and limitation?

What percentage of your time do you spend talking truth? What percentage of the time do you spend talking about illusions and pretense? What percentage of your time do you spend bad-mouthing yourself?

In addition, consider these questions:

-Do you speak about your feelings?
-Do you express boundaries, needs and wants?
-How do you speak? Strongly? Or with a quiet voice?
-Do you mostly talk? Or do you mostly listen?
-How do you feel after you speak?
-How do you present yourself?
-How do you use your voice? Do you use it to get things? Do you use it to express appreciation? Do you use it to complain?

Exercise #2:

Sing a song.

"Sing. Sing a song. Sing out loud. Sing out strong. Sing of good things, not bad. Sing of happy, not sad. Sing. Sing a song. Make it simple to last your whole life long. Don't worry that it's not good enough for anyone else to hear. Just sing. Sing a song."
-Karen Carpenter

Start vibrating the frequency of your own voice speaking/singing truth, love and joy to your cells!

Exercise #3:

Do the opposite of what you normally do:

- If you normally talk, then listen.
- If you normally listen, then talk.
- If you normally complain a lot, complain not at all.
- If you normally praise everything and everyone, be quiet (this might seem like a strange rule, but the addict is very sneaky and spends an exorbitant amount of time praising others in order to be liked and to get his needs taken care of)
- If you normally attack, then start to praise.
- If you normally give, then receive.
- If you normally receive, then give.
- If you are normally quiet, be loud.
- If you normally are loud, be quiet.

Day 11

Experimenting

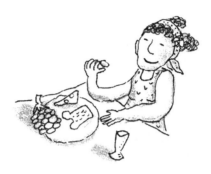

Today we are going to ask you to start disrupting your routine and start EXPERIMENTING.

Addicts like things to be a certain way. They like predictability. They know what is safe and stick with it.

Addicts want to be the best. Typically they find one area that works for them (most generous, most helpful, most caring) and then attempt to excel in this area to help give the impression that they are "normal" like everyone else.

The reason addicts do this is because they hate making mistakes or looking like fools. They can't stand to be vulnerable. So they do everything within their power to hold together an image of perfection, which usually means sticking with a certain routine.

Addicts are great performers! They like to know in advance what is going to happen so they can prepare for it. This is an attempt to put on a good face and show the world that they're okay, good, fine, and not a screwed up mess. SHOWTIME!

The only way to make sure everyone sticks to their part is to attempt to control the environment, to control all the variables.

To be Master of the universe!

Addicts are constantly busy to prevent getting off track. God forbid if there is a free moment when something unpredictable could occur!

There was a time in my life when I even tried to figure out in advance what I thought OTHER PEOPLE were going to do so I could be prepared! Talk about crazy. I not only tried to figure out what I would do and say, but I tried to figure out what everyone else would do and say. I thought about every possible scenario and what my reaction would be if it occurred. Talk about insane. I wanted to be several steps ahead of the game at all times. Talk about exhausting.

Today's lesson is about experimenting.

Experimenting!

Exercise #1:

SIT QUIETLY.

Be as quiet as possible. Let this quiet be your dedication. Be really quiet. Be still.

While in this stillness, ask yourself this question:
"How can I take care of myself in new ways?"

Exercise #2:

Do something different today; or differently!

If you are always busy, do nothing.
If you eat the same breakfast every morning, eat something different.
If you always eat at home, go eat out in a restaurant.
If you always eat out in restaurants, prepare a meal at home.
If your life is disciplined and organized, start disrupting it.
If your life is a mess, start being more organized.

If you always say "no!" to parties, say "yes!" to one.
If you always socialize with friends, then stay home to a quiet night of watching a movie or reading.
If you watch TV, then go outside instead.
If you are always busy with work, then make time for creativity.
If you always go to work at the same time, alter your schedule.
If you are always behind the computer, go buy a flower and plant it.

Do something different! *Experiment.*

This means taking a leap of faith. It takes trust. There is no right or wrong way to do this. Experimenting is like being in the science lab. You will make mistakes. It will be messy. Some new ways will work and other ways will be disastrous. That's the beauty of experimenting!

You'll learn as you go along.

Doing different things, or just doing things differently will be terrifying and exhilarating. It can be uncomfortable and scary as you start branching out into unknown territory. Like any journey or hike through the wilderness, you might start to sweat. Your hair might look a mess. You might lose your way, and you probably won't be looking your best.

But great news! You don't have to be perfect! You already are perfect as God created you! THIS IS YOUR LIFE. It doesn't have to look gracious. It just has to be authentic.

How are you spending your days? When you look back over your life, you'll realize it's the small moments that stand out like diamonds in their brilliance and simplicity.

Day 12

Blame and Shame

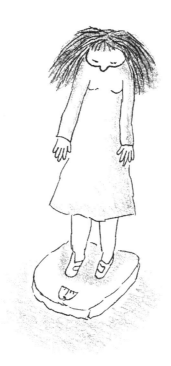

How do you treat yourself?

That's the big question of the day.

How do you treat yourself?
Are you yelling at yourself inside?
Are you blaming yourself constantly?
Are you full of shame?
Are you happy with what you accomplish or achieve?
Or are you immediately setting new goals and achievements?
Are you nice to yourself?
Do you celebrate your accomplishments?

The addict never gets it right. He is never good enough. He continually focuses on where he could have done it better. He is always looking for ways to improve himself, feeling full of blame and shame for not being perfect. He thinks he's not trustworthy.

He looks at what went wrong instead of what went right. He looks at the negative instead of the positive. He looks at his flaws instead of his better points. He strives for perfection and falls short time and time again. He is full of blame and shame for his sense of unworthiness.

Blame comes from an idea of deprivation.
Shame comes from secrecy.

Jesus tells us in *A Course in Miracles*:

"ONLY YOU CAN DEPRIVE YOURSELF OF ANYTHING. Do not oppose this realization, for it is truly the beginning of the dawn of light. Remember also that the denial of this simple fact takes many forms, and these you must learn to recognize, and oppose steadfastly and WITHOUT EXCEPTION. This is a crucial step in the re-awakening. The beginning phases of this reversal are often quite painful, for as blame is withdrawn from without, there is a strong tendency to harbor it within."
Urtext, Chapter 10, The Inheritance of God's Son

"If your brothers are part of you and you blame them for your deprivation, you are blaming yourself. Blame must be undone, NOT re-allocated."
Urtext, Chapter 10, The Inheritance of God's Son

"The body is the sign of weakness, vulnerability and loss of power."
ACIM, Chapter 20, The Vision of Sinlessness

"Perhaps there is fear and shame associated from a sense of inadequacy."
ACIM, Manual for Teachers, Should Healing be Repeated?

Blame and shame are attack. You're attacking yourself. Today we are undoing blame and shame, not re-allocating it.

One question should be asked:

"Is this what I would have, in place of Heaven and the peace of God? This is the choice you make. Be not deceived that it is otherwise. No compromise is possible in this. You choose God's peace or you have asked for dreams."
ACIM, Lesson 185, I want the Peace of God

You cannot enter God's presence when you attack, so today is the undoing of blame and shame, which ends all attack, and which allows you to enter into God's presence.

<u>Exercise #1:</u>

WRITE DOWN THE HIGHLIGHTS OF YOUR LIFE IN YOUR JOURNAL.
WRITE DOWN YOUR ACCOMPLISHMENTS.

Think back on your life and remember all the great things you have done.

Most addicts glaze right over their achievements. If they get five A's on their report card, they focus on the one B+ and beat themselves up over it for the next six months.

It's a fear of being ordinary. An addict wants to stand out as being special. He can't stand to have a minor role. He has high ideals and wants to be different, wants to be recognized and appreciated for his efforts.

He thinks he has to be the best to be loved.

The addict thinks BIG! He often has thoughts of grandiosity, but as well he is his own worst critic, his own harshest judge.

Today we ask you to accept the GLORY and RECOGNITION that is yours for all of your awesome accomplishments.

Today we ask that you accept the GRANDEUR that is your inheritance. The whole universe is rejoicing over your achievements and all the ways that you have been helpful, an inspiration, a guide, a light in the dark.

Exercise #2:

Plan a party for yourself to celebrate your achievements. Bring out the champagne. Bring out the bubbly.

Imagine you are a celebrity and this party is being thrown for you for all the amazing work you have done in your life. Imagine you are being given a lifetime achievement award for all your inspiring work. Celebrate your successes today!

Day 13

Dealing with tension

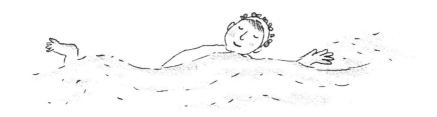

Tension. It's just a normal part of life, right?

Wrong.

"Tension is the result of a building-up of unexpressed miracle impulses."

Urtext, Chapter 1, Distortions of Miracle Impulses

Tension results when you are not expressing yourself. It occurs when you let things build up inside of you, and often results in an inability to move.

Tension is stagnant contained energy.

When you attempt to contain energy (as opposed to letting it flow), it causes all sorts of havoc.

Today's topic is: HOW TO DEAL WITH TENSION.

Since tension is "a building-up of unexpressed miracle impulses", trying to "think away" tension will get you nowhere.

You've got to start moving the energy. There is no other way. You must start communicating.

And here is where most addicts will begin to experience difficulty. Most addicts are afraid of movement and action. They are afraid of making a mistake. They are afraid of expressing themselves. So they bottle up everything inside and the result is TENSION.

Tension = Tense = Trapped.

You might feel trapped in your life, trapped in your relationships, trapped in your house, trapped in your body, trapped by your condition/addiction.

Tense.

Think about when you are tensing up.

We're asking you to come out of hiding. One of the best ways to start dealing with tension is to expose yourself.

I'll start. I'll go first. I haven't found the motivation to do any exercise lately.

I'm taking the tiniest baby steps. I haven't worked up to walking or running, but I do go outside now several times a day. I take breaks. I relax. I sit out in the sun. I call friends on the phone and tell them how I'm feeling. I'm more active. I'm more creative.

On most days lately, I feel gorgeous.

I'm being gentle with myself. I have a good steady pace. I don't beat myself up anymore. I'm not attacking myself for not getting it right. This is a huge miracle!! I might not have a perfect eating plan and I'm not losing weight at the moment, but I'm nice to myself now. That's a miracle.

I trust that the universe is helping me - that loving angels are everywhere - and that I simply have to keep following the path, knowing that healing is inevitable for me.

"All real pleasure comes from doing God's Will."
Urtext, Chapter 1, Distortions of Miracle Impulses

Opening up, releasing tension, allows the miracle to happen!

This 40-day Program might seem like hard work. And we know you're busy. But this is excavating and we didn't say it was going to be easy. Please just hang in there. Please just keep showing up every day.

Marielle and I, with your help and willingness, are going right in to gut out the big root that is causing all your problems. We are going to the source of the problem and not just working with symptoms.

And at the same time we hope you are enjoying these topics. We know we are pushing all your buttons. Good! We're thrilled! Having your buttons pushed is great news for us. It means a shift is occurring.

We could just offer another diet, but diets work as band-aids. *It Matters Totally* is not a band-aid solution. This is surgery. This is full-blown recovery from a lifetime of self-sabotage.

Here's a quick little personal story that might be helpful:

The Dandelion Flower: Getting out the Root

The other day I was out mowing grass because my whole front lawn was full of dandelions. I thought you could just chop off the yellow flowers and that would be that. WRONG! Have you ever looked close up at a dandelion? It is a bitch of a plant. It's got one big root with a whole cluster full of flowers and buds, some open, some closed. Within 30 minutes of mowing my entire front lawn, it was filled with dandelions again! I couldn't believe it. What?!?!?!?!

This reminds me of dieting. In the past, I would lose 10 pounds, and one week later, gain it all back, plus some. That's because I only chopped off the dandelion flower. I was only dealing with surface symptoms and that will never, ever, never work.

The only way really to get rid of the dandelion for good is to destroy the root. There is no other way.

And so it is with this work. We are not just working with your symptoms of overeating and addiction. We are going in to GUT out the root. It can seem difficult and brutal. We apologize. You asked for our help. You'll be laughing later in happiness when you realize your food addiction is gone, gone, gone.

There is more healing occurring now than you could ever imagine, and we love you for every step you take along the way. So let's deal with that tension!

Exercise #1:

Tense up your hands. Keep them tensed.

How does that feel? It's uncomfortable. After a couple of seconds you'll start to feel your heart working faster (and not in a good way). How long can you keep your hands tensed up in that position? A couple minutes at most? At a certain point, you can't stand it for another second and you let go. Your breathing returns to normal. *You let go.* You stopped tensing. After a few minutes tension becomes really painful. You can't stand it. It starts to cripple you.

Literally, tension will cripple you. It's energy that's not moving, and energy NEEDS to move. So first, you must become aware of the effects of tension in your life.

Recognize that you are bottling yourself up. If you're tense, you're not expressing yourself.

It's important to learn to LET GO. It's important to get the energy moving. It's important to start learning to express yourself.

Exercise #2:

When you are feeling tense, go do something completely different.

Move out of your space. Go into another room. Go outside. Go for a run. Walk. Stretch. Call a friend. Meet someone for a coffee. Go for a drive in your car. Take a bath. Drink a hot beverage. Get the energy moving.

Exercise #3:

Write in your journal: "BEAR THE TENSION."

You can handle much more than you think you can. When you absolutely cannot think you can bear the tension, remember that you can. Bear the tension. You are strong, powerful and you're never given more than you can handle.

Exercise #4:

Start expressing yourself. Reach out to others.

We'd like to invite you to start extending your love and light outwards, get the energy of yourself moving. You can start a blog (and I'll post a link). You can talk to strangers. You can reach out to help your neighbor. You can go to our website *It Matters Totally* (http://www. itmatterstotally.com) and write a comment about your experience with this program. You don't have to be brilliant. Just say what's going on with you. If you're scared, say it. If you're angry, say it. Be yourself. Be honest. Let it be messy. It doesn't matter. Make spelling mistakes. No one cares. You'll be surprised to find out that there are others in hiding who are waiting for someone to express/expose their most private thoughts and feelings.

I, Lisa, write daily blog articles about the workbook lessons of *A Course in Miracles* at a website called *Gorgeous for God* (http://www.GorgeousForGod.com), and you wouldn't believe how many people do not express themselves because they think they are the only ones who are "not getting it." I get emails from people who say they have wanted to write me for one year, but didn't because they're afraid of looking stupid. They think they should be happy (since *A Course in Miracles* promises happiness), and since they are embarrassed, miserable, lonely, sad, angry, depressed, tired, and bored, they think they must be doing something wrong. Instead of reaching out and asking for help, they stay quiet. They think they are the only ones having difficulty and they don't want to look stupid, so they say nothing. They just continue to be confused.

We're asking you to come out of hiding.

Day 14

Making mistakes

"If I had to live my life over again I'd dare
to make more mistakes next time."
-Nadine Stair

"Mistakes are the portals of discovery."
-James Joyce

Any artist will tell you that making mistakes is a necessary part of being creative. You can't make art without mistakes. They go hand-in-hand. You can't learn without making a mistake.

When you are ashamed of a mistake you are adding a mistake to a mistake! That's two mistakes instead of one!

Today we are going to turn your thinking upside down on the idea of making mistakes. You think it's best if you make as FEW mistakes as possible. We'd like you to start considering the possibility that making mistakes is a natural part of the discovery process. You don't have to be so careful anymore.

When you find a person who never makes a mistake, there you will find a person bound by hesitation and fear! I've seen it time and time again. A person who doesn't make mistakes is almost always playing it safe, and is stricken with fear about his own inferiority. He thinks it's best to walk cautiously to fool people into thinking he's perfect.

If you are not making a mistake at least a couple of times a week (preferably every day), then you are not living.

You are playing it safe, standing on the side-lines of life.

A Course in Miracles says that all mistakes have been corrected.

When you make a mistake, it simply calls for correction. That's all. Most addicts use their mistakes as another reason to savagely attack themselves and stay depressed.

Sometimes it's impossible to fix a mistake. It's impossible to turn back time. But how long are you going to attack yourself for something that happened and cannot be changed?

Don't spend too much time looking backwards. Just let mistakes become lessons and move on.

You might have accidentally killed someone while driving your car, or you hit a deer (or a dog or a cat) or someone was hurt while in your care. Maybe you said cruel things you regret? Maybe you never told someone you loved them and then they died before you had a chance to say all that was on your mind? Maybe you broke something that cannot be fixed? Maybe you hurt/abused someone because you just didn't know any better at the time?

Mistakes.

What was the lesson? How can you move forward?

"He has made a mistake, and must be willing to change his mind about it."
Urtext, Manual for Teachers, Should Healing be Repeated?

"Remember that all sense of weakness is associated with the belief that you are a body, a belief that is mistaken and deserves no faith."
Urtext, Lesson 91, Miracles are seen in Light

Mistakes call for correction. They call for forgiveness. You don't have to beat yourself up anymore. You can start being nice to yourself when you make a mistake.

Exercise #1:

Write down any mistakes you've made in your life. Forgive yourself now. Write them down and express your forgiveness as well.

Forgiving yourself for making mistakes takes infinite care, courage and gentleness. You really need to talk to yourself to imprint a new memory or instruction of kindness. GENTLENESS.

Exercise #2:

Make a declaration for yourself and write it down.
It could be something like this:

"I, Marielle, promise to support myself at all times. I give myself my freedom back to experiment and to try new things. I will be gentle with myself and allow myself to be lazy or just focus on myself whenever I need it. I will LOVE MYSELF through my mistakes. And TRUST MYSELF. I respect my desire to be free and I know that I have very good intentions for my life."

"I, Lisa, promise to try new things. I promise to take more risks in my life. I promise to be gentle with myself if I don't always "get it right." I will do the best that I can to be authentic, happy, playful, courageous, generous, passionate and always myself! I will *be* myself! That's my declaration. I will stop trying so hard to please other people. I will be myself. Those that like me will like me for who I am, as I am, flaws and all. I dedicate each day to being passionately alive, even if it means I make 100 mistakes!"

Exercise #3:

Get excited when you make a mistake!
It means you are growing. It means you are trying something new. It means you are taking new risks. Rejoice in your mistakes when they happen.

"Assert your right to make a few mistakes.
If people can't accept your imperfections, that's their fault."
-Dr. David M. Burns

"A life spent making mistakes is not only more honorable,
but more useful than a life spent doing nothing."
-George Bernard Shaw

"If you have made mistakes, even serious ones, there is
always another chance for you. What we call failure is not
the falling down, but the staying down."
-Mary Pickford

If you've made a mistake, don't stay down. Pick yourself up and move on. Rejoice.

WEEK 3
COMMUNICATION

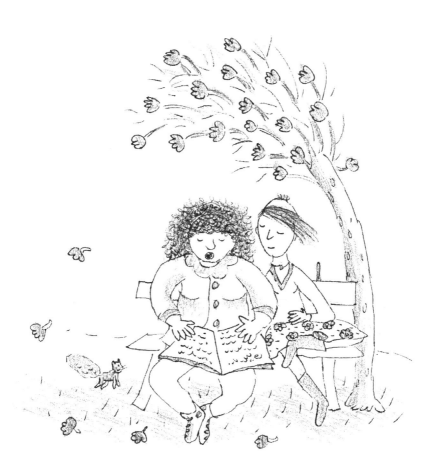

Day 15

Exposure

Welcome to Week 3!

The theme of this week is COMMUNICATION.

The topic for today is EXPOSURE.

This lesson is about learning to articulate exactly where you are, without hiding behind false certainty, happiness, kindness, goodness, or intelligence.

Today is a step toward learning to be yourself.

This lesson is also about HONESTY. Ask yourself the question: "How do I feel?"

Most addicts are not usually very honest with themselves. They feel tired, bored, or lonely but they keep these thoughts buried in a secret hiding place tucked behind a fake smile.

Are you tired, lonely, bored, angry, jealous, confused, or disappointed?

Did you do the exercise about LOOKING AT THE HIGHLIGHTS IN YOUR LIFE? Did you write down your achievements?

Most addicts when asked to name their achievements feel profound sorrow for a life that has passed them by. They feel they have nothing to show, and that it is too late for them to start living. With this recognition comes tremendous grief for the self that was abandoned.

A few years ago I cried and cried and cried for the precocious, creative, delightful, little girl named Lisa Lynn born in 1968 that I squashed. I put out the spark of joy in that little kid with all my rules of safety and precautions. At some point I started tiptoeing through life. It was like I was walking on eggshells. I looked before I made a move and then I walked with extreme caution. Don't upset anyone! Don't get mad! Don't cry! Don't raise your voice! Be a good little girl! Eat all your vegetables or you won't get any dessert!

It's time to start reclaiming your creative spark by starting to communicate your dreams, your goals, and your fears.

EXPOSURE!

Today it is time to start honoring your thoughts and exposing them.

Often, people are waiting for THE RIGHT TIME to get intimate with another person. They are waiting for right circumstances when they can let down their defenses and be vulnerable. They are waiting for a situation where they feel completely safe, cared for, loved and appreciated. They are waiting for an opening for someone to say "How are you feeling? Are you okay? Let's talk."

But here's the thing (you've probably already noticed): NO ONE EVER ASKS! There is never a safe moment. There is never a right time. Circumstances are never right for exposing your inner secrets.

So it's time to start communicating now. It's time to stop hiding.

Most addicts hide in isolation. They build a wall that they think keeps them safe. They don't like to bother other people and they don't like to be bothered themselves. Too much work! I'm too busy! I'm too boring! No one cares! I have nothing to say! My thoughts are meaningless!

But really, it's fear.

Most addicts try to work out their problems all by themselves. They try to fix themselves before they present themselves to their brother. They stay behind closed doors until they can present a great image to the world and to the neighbors.

I happen to think I am way too fat to be walking outside or riding a bicycle. I think I would look ridiculous. What will the neighbors think? But last night I was thinking about this topic of EXPOSURE and decided it was time to put on my sneakers and get on the bike and ride. It was so much fun! What was I waiting for? The seat needs to be adjusted but it was great, fantastic fun. I was waiting for a moment when I would feel safe (and fit and look good riding a bike); but I'd be waiting forever! I rode about a mile down the road when I passed a horse farm that I've always wanted to stop in. I saw four women outside the barn and I decided to stop.

EXPOSURE!

I had no reason to stop. I had nothing to say. I didn't have a plan. But I stopped anyway. It was so much fun! I met 4 women, 22 horses, 4 dogs and a kitten that fell completely in love with me. He was walking all over me. My own cat Enzo has been missing for 9 days and the kind of love I found at the horse farm was just what I needed!

Exposure.

All I said was "Oh, hi, I'm Lisa. I just wanted to introduce myself. I live down the road here. Just thought I'd stop in."

They were thrilled. Smiles and laughter all around. They brought out the sodas and we had a party.

It's time to start living.

"Do not hide suffering from His sight, but bring it gladly to Him."
ACIM, Chapter 13, The Fear of Redemption

Amazing, huh? Don't try to hide suffering from the Holy Spirit, just give it gladly to Him.

A Course in Miracles also says not to try to give yourself a miracle before going to the altar (to ask for a miracle). If you could give yourself a miracle, you wouldn't need to ask for one. Don't try to fix yourself up. Don't try to heal yourself. Don't try to clean up your addiction so that you can appear before God and then ask for help. Just show up.

Come with all of your addictions. Come with all of your grief. Come with your despair. Come in poverty. Come as you are and let yourself be healed.

Exercise #1:

What is today's topic? Exposure!

STOP PROCRASTINATING. It's time to start communicating what is going on with you. You can no longer wait until you feel safe.

Exercise #2:

Write or call on someone you can reach out to. You don't have to say anything important. Just start reaching out.

Exposure is about *vulnerability* and *availability*.
It takes courage to reach out to others.
It takes courage to make yourself available.

Exercise #3:

Be direct with others you interact with today. Ask for what you really want. Be specific.

Most addicts say things very indirectly. They want something but are afraid to ask for it directly. Instead they say "Oh, that coat is nice" while hoping that someone will get the hint and buy it for them.

Exposure is about honesty and no longer hiding behind false certainty. It is about bringing hidden secrets and desires out into the open sunlight for the world to see.

Day 16

Joining

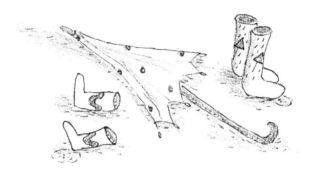

The topic of JOINING is twofold:

1. Joining with your brother
2. Joining with God

Isolation is first-nature for someone with food addiction.

Food addicts "join" with food. When they need comfort, solace, escape or relief they'd rather "meet" with something sweet, sugary, or salty than meet with a friend or God.

One food addict I know gained over 100 pounds in a year, and when I asked her about it she said, "When I'm fat, guys leave me alone. They don't bother me."

This is a woman who is really beautiful, and rather than learning how to deal with pick-up lines and men flirting with her, she has decided it is easier to make herself unattractive. She said to me: "I prefer to make love to a chocolate bar than to a man."

Meanwhile, she hates herself. She hates how she looks. She hates how she feels.

She wants love and appreciation but without all the demands that she thinks goes along with it.

She doesn't know how to join with someone. She doesn't know how to express her needs and boundaries. She wants to join with others but without everyone wanting something from her; without everyone expecting something of her.

She doesn't know how to let herself be loved.

She wants what we all want: to relax and be known. She wants to be loved and appreciated, but without all the demands and sacrifices of losing herself.

I've spent a lot of time with this girl, both at her lowest weight and at her heaviest weight, and the one consistent thing that has never changed is that she does not know how to relate to people. She's gorgeous - the kind of girl that takes your breath away - and you would expect she would be confident. Yet she is shy and insecure and wants only to be left alone. The only place she really feels truly safe is at home, near a box of cookies.

Now, I know this girl. She is gentle, sweet, kind, generous, a terrific cook, great with kids, loves animals, and has a wicked sense of humor. She is hilarious and fun to be with. When she's with me, she feels safe and is herself, which signifies that she does know how to join! When she's with me, there is an equal balance of sharing, laughter, honesty, and communication.

She knows she doesn't have to perform when she is with me. I know her. She knows me. And we understand each other. JOINING.

Joining means to meet in a space where you allow yourself to be yourself.

Joining means sharing, nurturing, no agenda, no plans, and no results.

Joining is the meeting of two minds as they share together in one bond, one purpose, one goal.

This can be "easier said than done" if you've never allowed yourself to stop performing. Most food addicts think they have to "do something" or "accomplish something" at all times. They think they have to be better than they really are. Food addicts can never just "be." They always want to be slightly different or a slightly better version of themselves.

Joining is seeing beyond separate interests. It is realizing that everyone is the same: everyone has the same needs, same fears, same goals, same wants. This is true joining. It is recognizing that you are One with all things, and realizing that your brother is exactly like you. It means you don't have to perform anymore. He's just as scared as you of being liked and judged. He wants only to be loved and appreciated.

To a food addict, friendships and love relationships = hard work.

You do all the work and someone else gets all the benefits, right?

Addicts think that relationships require lots of "doing" and "giving," so they are careful not to make any new commitments.

True joining is relaxation! It's a joy. It's fun. It's direct! It's nourishing! It will renew you, leaving you feeling creative and rejuvenated with passion.

Exercise #1:

Check in with yourself. Think about what it means to join with someone.

Ask yourself these questions:

> -How do I feel in joining with someone?
> -What emotions arise?

-Do I feel afraid, vulnerable, excited, or happy to join?
-Am I myself?
-Do I know what it means to be myself?

Exercise #2:

Organize a party/celebration with a friend to show your joy and healing.

This can be an invitation to have a coffee or a meal together. Whatever it is, make it special. This is a celebration for your dedication in this 40-day program. This is a great accomplishment and a great achievement. We want you to celebrate your healing with another person.

Exercise #3:

Start listening. Begin sharing your hopes and dreams with someone. Start allowing yourself to express yourself.

"What waits in perfect certainty beyond salvation is not our concern. For you have barely started to allow your first, uncertain steps to be directed up the ladder separation led you down. The miracle alone is your concern at present. Here is where we must begin. And having started, will the way be made serene and simple in the rising up to waking and the ending of the dream."

ACIM, Chapter 28, The Agreement to Join

Day 17

Prayer

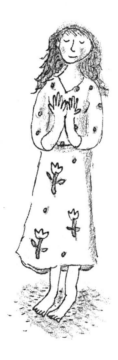

"Prayer changes things." –Emmet Fox

This is Week Three and the theme is COMMUNICATION. Prayer is the single most practical effective communication tool you can use to start creating with the Creator (who is your Father, by the way! He longs to give you everything)! Prayer is direct communication with God.

Most people use prayer as a way to "ask for something" and then they wonder why it doesn't seem to work. Prayer is a direct way to contact God. It's communication.

Here is a message from Jesus:

"You will see miracles through your hands through me. You should begin each day with the prayer 'Help me to perform whatever miracles you want of me today.'"
Urtext, Chapter 1, Introduction to Miracles

"PRAYER IS THE MEDIUM OF MIRACLES."
Urtext, Chapter 1, Introduction to Miracles, Principle #12

"The motivating factor is praying, or asking. What you ask for you receive. But this refers to the prayer of the heart, not to the words you use in praying."
ACIM, Manual for Teachers, What is the Role of Words in Healing?

VERY IMPORTANT: The words you use in prayer do not matter!

What matters is what is in your heart. What you ask for you receive. But this refers to the prayer of the heart, not to the words you use in praying.

So we want you to start practicing with prayer. Experiment. Find what feels right and good for you. You will begin TO FEEL IN YOUR HEART what a true prayer is. Play around with prayer until you find a method that brings peace to you and results in miracles.

**VERY IMPORTANT: PRAYER RESULTS IN MIRACLES.

"Miracles are natural. When they do not occur something has gone wrong."
ACIM, Chapter 1, Principles of Miracles, Principle #6

So if miracles are not occurring in your life, it's time to take a step back, stop what you are doing, and be willing to be shown what to do. The Holy Spirit is with you and He will tell you all you need to know.

"All miracles mean life, and God is the Giver of life. His Voice will direct you very specifically. You will be told all you need to know."
ACIM, Chapter 1, Principles of Miracles, Principle #4

I pray all day long. I talk to Jesus the way I would talk to my best friend. I recognize the necessity for help along this journey every day. I can't do this alone, but I'm not alone so I make use of the help that has been given to me! What a gift! I tell Jesus everything. I ask for everything. Sometimes I pray in writing. Sometimes I pray in silence, and sometimes out loud.

I pray before I go to bed. Usually I get on my knees to say a quick "goodnight and I love you" to God. But not always! I don't make it a ritual. Sometimes I am just too damn tired to get on my knees! So I crawl into bed and say a quick "thank you and I love you" while I'm turning out the light.

The form of the prayer doesn't matter! Thank the Lord. The only thing that matters is the sincerity in my heart while I am praying.

If I wake up in the middle of the night, my immediate response is "thank you, thank you, thank you, I love you." This is my prayer of the heart. What I've learned is that when I pray in this way I fall immediately back to sleep! Works like a charm! THANK YOU, THANK YOU, THANK YOU. THANK YOU GOD.

So today's topic on PRAYER is about learning to experiment and find what works for you.

Don't follow someone else's way to pray. Forget all the rules about praying. Find what works for you. Make it personal. Trust the guidance that is given to you.

What you are learning to do is to communicate with the invisible. There is a world beyond the world you experience with your five senses, and today you are going to begin interacting with that world. You do so through prayer. This is true communication.

Prayer is action of mind.

"The Holy Spirit is invisible, but you can see the results of His Presence and through them, you will learn that He is there. What He enables you to do is clearly not of this world, for miracles violate every law of reality as this world judges it. Every law of time and space, of magnitude and mass is transcended, for what the Holy Spirit enables you to do is clearly beyond ALL of them. Perceiving His results, you will understand where He must be, and finally KNOW what He is."

ACIM, Chapter 12, Looking Within

Exercise #1:

Sit in your place and enjoy it. Slow down. Stop rushing. Relax. There is a place in your mind where true communication happens, a place where you can be inspired. Know. Listen. Talk. Ask. Know that you are in the Presence of God. Your requests are being heard and answered.

Exercise #2:

Write a specific prayer and keep it on your night-table or put it in a box.

-What do you pray for?
-How do you pray?

Exercise #3:

Experiment with prayer. There is no right or wrong way to pray, but you will know when something is working for you.

Day 18

Standing in your own certainty

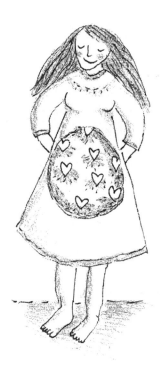

The mass majority of people have no idea what it means to stand in their own certainty. Most people are filled with self-doubt and so they look to other people for references and cues about their next steps.

Most people second-guess everything they do. They start to take a step in one direction and then they pull back in fear and doubt.

To stand in your own certainty means to make a decision and follow through with action. It means to stop waiting for something to happen. It means saying: "I AM GOOD ENOUGH. I AM GOING TO DO THIS."

I CAN DO THIS!

Have you ever watched dancers on a stage? Professional dancers dance in their own certainty. They stand in their own light. For all they care, they could be the only dancer on the stage. They know the steps by listening to the music and they give it 100%. They give it their all. They give it their best.

They are present, focused and graceful. They make dancing look easy.

Amateur dancers dance by watching others and trying to follow along. They are cautious and it shows. They are always a half-step behind. Their foot doesn't move until they see someone else's foot move. They are awkward and clumsy. They make dancing look difficult. Have you ever been in an audience and witnessed this? It throws off the whole performance.

But when each dancer is standing in his own certainty, dancing in his own light, the performance is a brilliant work of art. It's memorable, mesmerizing, inspiring and beautiful.

Each day is meant to be this way for you when you begin standing in your own certainty.

If you want your life to change (and most food addicts do), you must be willing to stop scattering your energy. To see change, you must change something you do every day. You must stop waiting for people to change or for circumstances to change. *YOU* MUST CHANGE.

You must do at least one thing differently if you expect to change. There is no other way. No "miracle" is going to save you. You determine what your life becomes by your thoughts and actions.

Exercise #1:

Write down your priorities.

-What is important to you?
-Is this list of priorities consistent with your life as it is now?
-What is your #1 priority?

For example:

If taking care of yourself is your #1 priority, does your life reflect this?
If spending time with your family is your top priority, do you spend
time each day with your family? Or do you spend most of your time
at work? If knowing God is your #1 priority, do you spend time with
Him each day?

Exercise #2:

What is one small specific action step you can take today to stand in
your own certainty?

You have to determine your priorities first before you can decide what
specific action step you are going to take. This lesson is about getting
clear, becoming focused, standing in the spotlight and knowing what
you want. Today's topic requires action.

It requires your getting clear on ONE SMALL SPECIFIC ACTION
STEP YOU CAN TAKE TODAY.

It is about taking your place in the universe.

You move, and then everything else moves with you.

This is a difficult lesson to do. At the time of writing this, I'm all over
the map. My energy is scattered all over, and as a result, I'm feeling
a bit frantic. I had guests in the B & B this weekend (8 adults) from
Friday afternoon to Monday morning, which was awesome terrific
fun, and now my attention is being pulled in 10 different directions.
I am not sure what I should do first. I have no idea what my priorities
are. My gut instinctual reaction is to do only what is in front of me for
today (laundry, make beds, do dishes, write blog posts, create a new

audio, do a radio show at 2pm), but today's topic is really an invitation TO LOOK AT THE LARGER PICTURE.

Relax. Breathe. Focus.

What's important to you? What are your priorities? LOOK AT THE OVERALL LARGER PICTURE. STEP BACK. What is important to you on a larger scale?

What is one small specific step you can take today?

The only way for me to accomplish this is to take 10 minutes for myself and go sit on the couch with pen and paper to come into my own certainty. This requires a conscious decision to forget everything else (just for 10 minutes!)

"But I don't have 10 minutes! I'm frantic! I've got 30 things that need to get done today! I don't have time for 10 minutes! Rush! Rush! Rush!"

Exercise #3:

Realize that all time is yours. Own that time.
Now do this with space.
Realize that all space is yours. Own that space.

You'll begin to feel yourself relax when you realize you don't have to do everything right now. You don't even have to do everything today. Or even this week. When you write down your priorities, you will realize there are some things in your life that you don't have to do at all anymore!

This lesson makes me happy. All time is mine. All space is mine. I have 10 minutes. In fact, I have 30 minutes. In fact, I have all day if I want. I can go sit on the couch (or outside) and reflect on what is important to me. The dishes and the laundry can wait.

Congratulations!

Day 19

Setting intentions

Most people think of intentions as goals to be achieved, and that's not what we are talking about here today.

Setting intentions is about aligning yourself with your priorities and remembering what is important to you.

Setting intentions is about setting the tone for your day at the beginning of the day.

You have been setting goals your entire life. You have succeeded and failed. Most food addicts are driven, determined super-achievers. "It is my intention to stick with this food plan/diet no matter what!" We all know the story. Most food addicts can go on a water fast for a week, no problem. I ate nothing but raw food for six months. Easy! I lost 40 pounds in 3 months. Effortless!

But then what happens when determination starts to slide a little?

We all know the answer. You wind up back where you started, and usually just a little bit worse. Once I started eating regularly again I gained 60 pounds (the 40 I'd lost in 3 months, plus 20 more). I would have been better off if I had never done it in the first place.

So Setting intentions is NOT the same as goal-setting. Setting an intention will give you IMMEDIATE RESULTS, in this very day.

It is my intention to be Gorgeous for God ... and so I am.
It is my intention to live my life on purpose ... and so I do.

IT IS WRITTEN.

It is my intention to have fun every day and to make that a priority.

It is my intention to be happy, free, joyous and live a creative life doing work I love.

It is my intention to take care of myself, to be authentic and express my needs and wants.

It is my intention to inspire people to know themselves as God created them... perfect.

It is my intention to focus on the positive and forget about the negative.

It is my intention to choose gratitude over grievances.

See the difference?

It is my intention to honor my word and follow through with my commitments.

"Intent is a force that exists in the universe. When sorcerers (those who live in Source) beckon intent, it comes to them and sets up the path for attainment, which means that sorcerers always accomplish what they set out to do."
-Carlos Castaneda

!!!!!!!!

Amazing, right?

"Sorcerers always accomplish what they set out to do." -Carlos Castaneda

And so it is with you. You are a miracle worker. You are healed and you can heal. You can have anything you want. You are a sorcerer when you make a decision to live in Source. There is nothing in all the world that can stop you from accomplishing all you set out to do.

Wayne Dyer wrote a great book called *The Power of Intention* and in it he says: "Imagine that intention is not something you do, but rather a force that exists in the universe as an invisible field of energy."

So today's topic is really about aligning yourself with a force that exists in the universe.

If you have been dieting (obsessing about food) your whole life so that you could be beautiful and start living your life, then a great intention is to be beautiful and start living your life. TODAY. That is setting an intention. You intend it and automatically it becomes true. Being beautiful and energetic comes from within, as does everything. The experience is available to you today.

Exercise #1:

Look at your priority list from yesterday. Celebrate that you are getting clear about what is important to you.

Yesterday we asked you to write down your priorities. Did you do that? If not, please take time to make your list today. Your healing cannot occur until you start realizing what is important to you. You need to know your priorities, and until then you will feel you are being pulled in 10 different directions.

Once you know your priorities, everything else falls easily into line. You might think your job is your #1 priority until you realize that your child or marriage is the most important thing of all. Your #1 priority might be taking care of yourself and doing work you love. If that is the case, then you will stop doing things you don't love! As you get clear you will begin to shift your energy to nurture those things that are at the top of your list.

Exercise #2:

What are your intentions for today? Write them down in your journal.

What are your intentions for your life? Write them down in your journal.

Marielle and I were talking about the trap of trying to give up sugar and the temptation to start dieting/binging again.

Remember... we are in the middle of the desert and the devil will come to tempt you! So be aware when it happens.

Originally it was my "intention" to quit sugar. I had identified sugar as my personal poison. So I made a huge sweeping declaration: "I'm giving up sugar!" But five seconds later, all I was able to think about was how much I wanted sugar. This happens because *sugar* is NOT a personal poison... judgment is!

So a good intention would be: "I intend not to judge myself today. I intend to love myself and to be in a state of gratitude. I intend to treat myself with kindness."

Exercise #3:

Feel the difference between making an "intention" based on restriction versus making an intention based on abundance.

Exercise #4:

Think of ways you can rejuvenate so that you feel young again.

Day 20

Friendship based on freedom

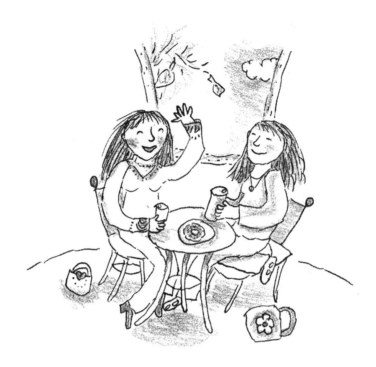

A friend is someone you know, like and trust.

The big question of the day is:
ARE YOU A FRIEND TO YOURSELF?

Do you KNOW yourself?
Do you LIKE yourself?
Do you TRUST yourself?

Friendship based on freedom first starts with you becoming a friend
to yourself.

Jim Morrison, lead singer of The Doors, says: "A friend is someone who lets you have total freedom to be yourself."

That's true. Now here's a question: Do you allow yourself to have total freedom to be yourself?

We are flipping the idea of friendship around here so that you begin to honor and nurture your relationships:

-your friendship with God
-your friendship with Jesus
-your friendship with yourself
-your friendship with others

A Course in Miracles says you have "An Appointed Friend", and it's you. Your appointed friend is Christ Who lives in you, who is You!

God has appointed a friend to you! Isn't that exciting? He has given you a constant friend and companion who will never, ever leave you! You're never alone! Your best friend goes with you always. Your Appointed Friend will always be there for you, ready to give you everything.

This is the most important friendship to begin nurturing. This is the reason it is so important to start taking care of yourself, to start LIKING yourself, to begin trusting yourself, and to start doing nice things for yourself.

Most friendships are created to supply a lack. They are the search for completion. You look for in another what you think you are lacking in yourself. You think a friend or a lover can fulfill you, complete you, and make you happy, and this is the whole problem of separation.

Friendship WITHOUT freedom is usually based on one of the following two things:

1. Being a caretaker, trying to get people to like you, love you, appreciate you.

2. Being needy and helpless and trying to get people to listen, support and help you.

This is not friendship. This is attack.

Friendship based on freedom is where you do work on yourself FIRST. You find your own completion and wholeness, and then you extend it in joy and generosity.

In a place of completion, you are no longer looking TO GET. You allow everyone to be exactly as they are, and you suddenly start to relax and have fun (miracle of all miracles!)

My whole life I wanted to be liked by others. I wanted to fit in. I craved friendship. I NEEDED it. I was the kind of girl that needed a relationship at all times. But I could never believe that someone actually wanted to hang out with me. It was a constant surprise to me that people liked me. Whenever someone told me they thought I was funny, smart or beautiful, I thought they must be blind!

I never thought I was good enough.

How could anyone want to be my friend? I thought I was full of flaws, insecure, shy, awkward and boring! I couldn't imagine why anyone would choose me for a friend.

And so when it actually happened, I didn't trust it. I thought I had to put on a show. I thought I had to perform because obviously there had been a huge mistake in the accounting office, right?? Someone wanting to be my friend must be a glitch, and I would soon be discovered for the loser that I actually was. They'd realize they'd make a huge mistake and then move on to more interesting, attractive people.

I didn't like myself so I couldn't imagine anyone else liking me either.

Total hatred of myself. I hated every aspect about myself, but I so needed to be loved! So I ate. Food was my friend. It comforted me, never judged me, and I never had the feeling that food would leave me. It was always there for me, my constant soothing companion, until it started becoming my enemy!

I was very relieved when I found *A Course in Miracles*. It gave me a new reference, a new way of thinking. It brought Jesus back into my life.

I stopped caring so much about other people's opinions because suddenly I had a Friend who loved me, no matter what I looked like, no matter what I did, no matter my mistakes! Talk about relief!

Once I started to enjoy my own company, a miraculous thing happened: lots of people suddenly wanted to be my friend!

Oh, the paradox!

When I stopped caring about being popular and well-liked, authentic and genuine friendships started coming my way. I no longer had to seek people out. They found me! I no longer had to perform. I knew these friends liked me for me.

Just for fun, I found some great quotes on friendship:

"A friend may well be reckoned the masterpiece of Nature."
-Ralph Waldo Emerson

"My friends are my estate."
-Emily Dickinson

"My best friend is the one who brings out the best in me."
-Henry Ford

"I do not wish to treat friendship daintily, but with the roughest courage. When they are real, they are not glass threads of frost work, but the solidest thing we know."
-Ralph Waldo Emerson

"Many people will walk in and out of your life, but only true friends will leave footprints in your heart."
-Eleanor Roosevelt

You are one of the best things that's ever happened to me. You're my love and my best friend. And every day that goes by, it seems like I discover something new about you to love. It's incredible to me how one person can make such a big difference in my life. You touch my heart in a way I never knew before. I discover something new about you to love. It's incredible to me how one person can make such a big difference.
-Author Unknown

Exercise #1:

Write in your journal the qualities you look for in a friend.

Do you display these qualities in yourself?

Exercise #2:

Give yourself the gift of your own friendship.

It is powerful to become your own best friend. This is total freedom. You no longer need to be caught in the trap of a search for completion. Supply your own lack! Love yourself as only a real best friend would. Be your own best friend!

Day 21

Asking for help

Here is a tough one for all the addicts of the world: Asking for help!

Are you always taking control?
Do you try to carry all the responsibility?
Do you share in the burden with others? Or carry it by yourself?
Do you try to solve problems on your own?
Do you ask for help only when there is no other alternative?
Would you rather give up than ask for help?
Do you drop hints instead of being specific about what you want/need?
Do you think that ignoring a problem will make it go away? (or that someone else will take care of it eventually?)

Asking for help is a communication skill.

We are on the last day of Week 3 and the theme is COMMUNICATION.

A big part of communication is asking for help, and most addicts are without any experience in this department. They want to do everything by themselves for a number of reasons:

- They don't want to bother or inconvenience anyone.
- They think the job gets done best if they do it alone.
- They don't want anyone to think they are weak or helpless.
- They have a fear of joining (which is ultimately a fear of communication).

So today's topic is really about learning a new communication skill: Asking for help!

Asking for help = Communication.
Asking for help = Being Connected.
Asking for help = Joining.
Asking for help = Trusting.
Asking for help = Exposure.

You probably never thought of it that way. You probably have only thought of "Asking for help" as weakness, neediness, inconvenience, hassle, and loss of control.

What if you ask someone for help and they want to do it their way???

Arrrrrggggggggggghhhhhhhhhhhhhhhh! An addict's worst nightmare is loss of control!

What if someone says "no"?

What if someone realizes that you're not rich, smart, certain, confident or brave?

Better to just do everything by yourself, right? Better to uphold the appearance that you get along just fine on your own.

But at what price do you pay?

My big excuse was that it was easier for me to do the job alone than to try to explain what needed to be done.

Also, I was constantly afraid someone was going to give me a lecture on "the way I was living my life." It seemed best just to keep all the windows and doors shut in my life and not let anyone get too close to look in on the particulars (that I didn't have money, that I was struggling with a food addiction, and that I was mostly really lazy).

Certainly, it was best just to keep up the appearance that I was smart, beautiful and energetic and could do everything by my self! And as well, better to exhaust myself with non-stop work and constant rushing than to ask for help! Better to have stress, anxiety and high blood pressure than to allow myself to be vulnerable, right?

This is the insanity of addiction. I'd rather harm myself than ask for help.

But here's the thing: I LOVE IT WHEN SOMEONE ASKS FOR MY HELP!

I love it, I love it, I love it. It makes me feel useful and wanted. It gets me moving. I love being able to help my brother. I love giving and I love the moment when someone calls me on the phone or emails me and says "I need your help." All my senses come alive! I spring to action!

Realizing how happy I was when someone asked for my help, it became clear to me that by NOT asking my brother for help I was denying him a huge gift.

People love to help! They do!

And if they are busy, they will say no. Plain and simple. But most everyone loves that moment when they realize they are needed. The Power of Asking!

Jesus says: "Ask and receive."

"Ask for my help to roll away the stone."

The other great benefit of asking for help is that you tap into feminine energy, which is completely different than masculine energy.

On the journey home to God you must begin to merge these two energies, balance them, integrate them to become One rather than be so heavy-handed on one side.

Masculine Energy is:

Assertive
Logical
Hunting
Doing
Controlling
Aggressive
Thrusting
Rushing
Organizing
Striving
Protecting
Survival

Feminine Energy is:

Intuitive
Receiving
Creative
Nurturing
Receptive
Soft
Allowing
Being
Surrender
Trusting
Feeling

Today there is only ONE EXERCISE and it's a doozy.

Exercise #1:

ASK FOR HELP.

Ask someone for help today even if you think you can do it on your own.

Have fun tapping into female energy! You'll love it. Ask for help.

WEEK 4
CREATIVITY

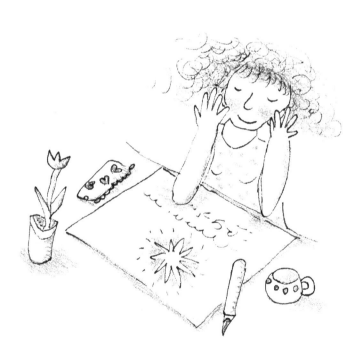

Day 22

Playing

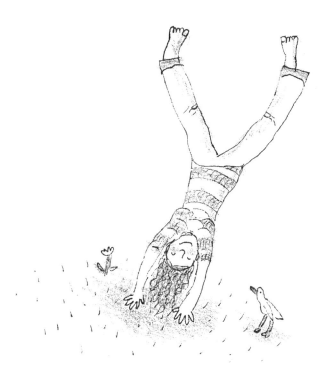

Playing is about becoming little children.

"Verily I say unto you, Except ye be converted, and become as little children, ye shall not enter into the kingdom of heaven."
-Matthew 18:3

"'Except ye become as little children' means that unless you fully recognize your complete dependence on God, you cannot know the real power of the Son in his true relationship with the Father."
ACIM, Chapter 1, The Escape from Darkness

Playing is not a luxury. Playing is a NECESSITY if you are to begin to know the Power that has been given to you by God. There is no other way.

"The basic decision of the miracle-minded is NOT to wait on time any longer than is necessary."
 Urtext, Chapter 1, Distortion of Miracle Impulses

So we want you to start playing today.

We want you to dedicate every day to playing from now on.

You are a holy CHILD of God. Children love to play!

"Child of God, you were created to create the good, the beautiful, and the holy."
 Urtext, Chapter 1, Distortion of Miracle Impulses

Remember when your mother or father used to scream at you to "GO OUTSIDE AND PLAY"! They weren't giving you an option. You didn't have a choice in the matter. It was a command and a demand.

This is today's instruction: START PLAYING!

Most people (especially spiritual seekers) are serious individuals, doing serious adult-like things: teaching, counseling, making money, taking responsibility, and "saving the world."

Salvation is not serious business.

I love to play. I like to have fun. Last year I decided to play that I was rich and that I was going to buy a house. I did this during a time when I didn't have a dime to my name. I always wanted a house but I never had any money, so I didn't even dare to look. But then one day I thought: well maybe there is something to all this Law of Attraction stuff. What harm is there in looking? So I called realtors and looked at magnificent houses and played the game of what it would be like to live in these houses. It was pure fun: long leisurely afternoons that stand out like bright sunbeams in my memory.

And now, today, I live in one of those houses.

Playing!

Another example: I love wedding dresses. They are so beautiful. Who can resist? So I try them on for fun at Goodwill. Who cares? All my friends think it's hilarious. "Oh, there goes Lisa again, trying on wedding dresses." And we all burst out laughing hysterically and before you know it: all my friends are trying on dresses. In a short time, all the customers in the shop are laughing along with us and occasionally, trying on dresses too! Playing is contagious! Suddenly everyone wants in on the game. I get the feeling that lots of girls secretly want to try on wedding dresses, but feel it's inappropriate unless you are engaged and getting married. Go ahead! You have permission! Who cares if you don't have a boyfriend? Playing dress-up with friends is a great way to spend the day.

"Salvation can be thought of as a game that happy children play. It was designed by One Who loves His children, and Who would replace their fearful toys with joyous games which teach them that the game of fear is gone. His game instructs in happiness because there is no loser. Everyone who plays must win, and in his winning is the gain to everyone ensured. The game of fear is gladly laid aside when children come to see the benefits salvation brings."

"You who have played that you are lost to hope, abandoned by your Father, left alone in terror in a fearful world made mad by sin and guilt, be happy now. That game is over. Now a quiet time has come in which we put away the toys of guilt, and lock our quaint and childish thoughts of sin forever from the pure and holy minds of Heaven's children and the Son of God. We pause but for a moment more, to play our final happy game upon this earth. And then we go to take our rightful place where truth abides and games are meaningless."
    ACIM, Lesson 153, In my defenselessness my safety lies.

Wow. Amazing. Life is meant to be a happy game.

"We pause but for a moment more, to play our final happy game upon this earth. And then we go to take our rightful place where truth abides and games are meaningless. So is the story ended"
ACIM, Lesson 153, In my defenselessness my safety lies

So is our healing accomplished!

<u>EXERCISE #1:</u>

Think back to when you were a kid.
What kinds of things did you love to do?
Write in your journal about that child.

<u>Exercise #2:</u>

Delight in small pleasures

Don't turn playing into another serious thing you have to do as a responsibility. This is about having fun. Borrow a child for the afternoon (do you have any idea how many parents would love a break?). Go play with the neighbors' pets. Go to a local toy store or to the movies. Dance in the living room. Play your records. Start "saving your allowance" to buy something you really, really, really want. Remember what it was like to save your allowance? For me, the anticipation was as exciting as buying the thing itself.

<u>Exercise #3:</u>

Find a playmate.

This exercise is crucial. You need playmates. It's more fun when you have a "partner-in-crime"; a friend to laugh with, scheme with, dress up with, and to bounce off your crazy ideas.

For children, there is no limitation. You can be anything you want. You can be a dancer, a doctor, a scientist, a princess, an explorer, or an astronaut who travels to the stars. You can be a writer, a teacher, an artist, or a superhero with awesome powers.

You can be whatever you want.

You can do whatever you want.

You can have whatever you want.

In the realm of mind/imagination, the possibilities are endless. You are a Child of God, a priceless part of His Kingdom, which He created as part of Him.

Day 23

Recovering your sense of wonder

The mass majority of people take everything for granted.

Do you realize what a miracle it is that we can communicate with each other? Have you ever looked at it? Thought about it?

It's a miracle on a scale so magnificent that I don't know what to do! To be IN A STATE OF WONDER is to be in A STATE OF INSPIRATION. To be inspired is to be in Spirit.

You start seeing things through the eyes of Christ. You realize everything is a miracle.

Your relationships are a miracle. Your life is a miracle. *You* are a miracle!

You stop taking things for granted. Your senses come alive.

Think about something as "basic" as communication. You have thoughts in your mind. That alone is a miracle. Then you open your mouth and sound vibrations organize the thoughts. These vibrations pass through the air, the phone, the computer and someone else is able to understand what you are thinking. Amazing. How does that work??

If that doesn't leave you in a state of awe, I don't know what will.

How does the internet work??? I have no idea, but it's crazy, splendid, beautiful and thrilling!

My thoughts are coming through my finger tips right now, typing on a keyboard, and I can push a button and in less than 30 seconds, no matter where you live, you will all know what I am thinking. That's amazing!

It's WONDER-full!

Your body is an awesome machine. It functions perfectly: breathing, heart beating, digesting, cleansing. It moves you through time and space! You complain about your body when in truth, it's spectacular!

Have you ever taken the time to appreciate your body?

Have you given thanks and gratitude for your ability to walk, talk, think, eat, love, feel and create?

Look at the cell phone. A piece of plastic and metal with the ability to pinpoint with perfect precision anyone, anywhere in the world. You can live on the other side of the Atlantic or the Pacific Ocean and it doesn't matter. I can still locate you by pushing some buttons.

This is what it means to recover your sense of wonder.

You probably take it for granted that you can get on an airplane and fly or get in your car and drive.
It's a miracle!

How about the wonder of electricity, refrigeration, heat, indoor plumbing and running water?

Sheer craziness, insanity, and brilliance!

I spend half my day in shock, excitement, and joy over simple things. I used to take everything for granted, and now I take nothing for granted.

A lot of people talk about the Law of Manifestation and they are upset that they are not good at it. But you are great at manifestation!! You have manifested everything that is in your life right at this very moment. You manifested your child, your car, your house, your relationships, your job, and all of nature outside your window. You have manifested a whole world! You manifested me and Marielle. You manifested the book you are reading these words on. Everything that you see, you brought into existence!

RECOVER YOUR SENSE OF WONDER!

To recover your sense of wonder is to begin to look at everything with new eyes.

To re-cover means to "get back, regain something lost or taken away, restore a former condition, regain strength, composure, balance."

This is a journey to find yourself; to become connected again to Spirit.

To recover your sense of wonder is to get excited and happy about things you once took for granted.

A cup of coffee. It amazes me. It includes Columbia or Italy and the people who pick coffee beans for a living, the factories that bag it, the truck drivers who transport it, as well as the airplanes that get it to the U.S., and the shop owners. And more.

An apple. A banana. Asparagus. Sugar. Chocolate. Flour. Do you ever think about where they come from? They include all of nature: the sun, the soil, and the rain. They include the energy of those individuals who got them to your doorstep.

Recovering your sense of wonder.

You're not "doing" anything. You simply begin looking at things differently.

To be in a state of wonder is to be in a constant presence of being and alertness.

EVERYTHING IS A GIFT.

This lesson is an invitation to awaken your senses.

Exercise #1:

Write down the wonders in your life.

Exercise #2:

Write down inspirational thoughts and quotes. Put them in a place where you will see them.

Exercise #3:

Take a walk in nature. Go outside. Find treasures to keep: a stone, a flower, a stick, a penny, a piece of paper (which formally you looked upon as trash). Paper is a miracle!! It comes from trees!

Exercise #4:

Celebrate your body. Take time today to give thanks for all the ways it functions perfectly. Be in a state of wonder about your arms, your legs, your heart, your mind, your sense of smell, taste, touch, sound, and sight.

Day 24

Movement of energy

This lesson has nothing to do with the body.

This is NOT an action lesson because energy moves automatically when you let go of your tight control.

Today's lesson is about surrender and allowing the energy of you to move to where it wants to go.

Almost all addicts are very tightly-strung, tightly-wrapped, and stressed-out. They like things a certain way. They like the predictable and familiar. They like routines, even as they wish their life was more exciting and spontaneous.

Holding yourself together as a perfect picture of "okay-ness" is an attempt to hold energy in one place. But energy likes to move! It loves to flow! A river does not stand still. The wind cannot be limited. The sun shines everywhere.

You cannot contain light, energy and Spirit. If you attempt to limit Spirit, the body starts to shut down. It has no choice!

Have you ever had a plant in a pot that was too small? Have you watched what happens? It stops growing and eventually it begins to die. It needs a bigger pot. The roots need more space.

And so it is with you. You cannot be contained. You need new spaces. That's the reason we had you create a space for yourself at the beginning of this 40-day course: so that you begin widening your range of experiences.

Back when I started this 40-day program I was very much a home-body. I mostly stayed in my bedroom. Then I created a space for myself in the library. It was sunnier and brighter and the Spirit of me was immensely pleased. After that, I started branching out to the dining room, and then the living room. Then I opened all the doors and windows, and now I spend a lot of time outside.

Movement of energy.
New spaces.
New faces.

If the energy of you wants to move to wider spaces and you don't let it, you will start to get sick. Guaranteed.

It takes the form of "letting yourself go."

You stop caring. You start to atrophy, with degeneration or decline from misuse. Sound familiar?

Have you stopped caring? Have you started to let yourself go?

If you allow the mind to get weak and lazy, your body starts to get weaker. When you stop caring about yourself, your body begins to decline.

Overweight bodies, sickness and old age are all symptoms of stuck energy.

Stuck energy is resistance, not caring, control.

You know when you are stuck. You can't move. You don't want to get out of bed. You feel bad. You feel tired. Your movements are slow and heavy. You don't feel like writing in your journal. You don't feel like talking to anyone. You feel overwhelmed, afraid and bored.

It means you're stuck. It's a desperate place to be. You start to believe this is part of life. You start to accept your stuck condition as normal. It's not normal! It's what death is. You're dying a slow death.

Energy needs to move. You can't contain it. You can't keep it limited. Certainly, you can attempt to stay small and limited but you're only hurting yourself because energy affects the system it lives in. You can't escape by hiding.

"The peace of God can never be contained. Who recognizes it within himself must give it."
Urtext, Workbook Lesson 188, The peace of God is shining in me now.

Are you holding yourself together?
Or are you letting energy flow through you?

Movement of Energy is about giving yourself a bigger pot to grow in. It's about widening the space. It's about broadening your mind.

First you move the mind and then the body follows naturally.

The Light is always coming through you, but most people stop it at the body level. They don't let it flow. They try to control their experiences. Too scary to talk to your brother! Too terrifying to express yourself! Too intimate to expose your thoughts!

Most addicts push, pull, plot, plan, and manipulate in an attempt to move the body. They use diets, fasting, exercising, working harder and smarter, and writing "to-do" lists.

But the body is nothing! It does not exist! It is impossible to change the body through behavioral attempts, except for temporarily. And these temporary changes are random in effect. They never last (as you probably have already realized).

There is no change possible at the behavioral level. None. Zero. All real change happens at the level of mind.

Change your mind and the body will change automatically.

Exercise #1:

Go somewhere you have never been before.

Exercise #2:

Do something you have never done before.

These exercises start in your mind. Think about someplace you've never been before.

Maybe you have never been happy. Go there.

Do you say "sorry" all the time? Go to where apologies are not needed.

Do you shut yourself off from people? Then pick up the phone and call someone. Go there.

Maybe you have never been financially responsible? That would be a place you've never been before, and a great place to go.

Do you rush all the time? Then rest is movement of energy for you. Go there. Take a nap. Relax on the couch. Read an enjoyable book for the fun of it.

Remember, you are not moving the energy, you are allowing the energy to move you. This is what it means to "do nothing." You let the Spirit move you. *Your* job really is to stop controlling and to stop trying to contain the energy.

Once you relax and trust, the energy will start moving you. You will simply go where it takes you. You let Him (the energy of Love) lead the way.

Paul in a letter to the Corinthians (15:52) in the bible says "In a moment, in the twinkling of an eye... we shall be changed" and that's absolutely true. Transformation is guaranteed. You'll start to realize that you are doing nothing at all, except giving a little willingness to allow yourself to be changed. There is a Power in you that begins to move you, change you, heal you. When you start relaxing in Spirit, you will see that the energy of you moves, and then the body automatically follows.

So you can stop trying to move the body now.

Instead, relax and trust. Let the energy flow to wherever it wants to go, allowing yourself to be lifted and carried by God Himself.

Day 25

Flexibility/Improvisation

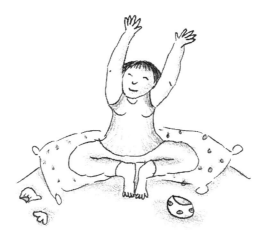

Flexibility is the key to seeing miracles.

This is a fact.

Why is this so? Think about it. In order to see a miracle, that means something would have to change in your life, right? If your life is not a miracle now, then in order for it to be a miracle it means that something unexpected and spontaneous must occur for you. Correct? And then you would say: "IT'S A MIRACLE!"

Which would mean that something new happened for you.

To be flexible means to:

> -bend without breaking
> -be willing to yield
> -be responsive to change

To be flexible means to allow yourself to flow and bend.

Flexibility requires that you be alert, present and open to new possibilities.

It means you have a willingness to drop your plans (diets, goals, agenda) when necessary.

Improvisation is about being spontaneous and responsive to your immediate environment, constantly looking for clues and ways to be in harmony with others. It is making, creating or inventing with what is given; with what is directly in front of you.

Inflexibility on the other hand is rigidity, unwillingness, resistance to being bent. It is not permitting change or variation; unalterable.

Are you flexible?
Is your day flexible?
Is your schedule flexible?
Is your eating flexible? Or do you always eat the same foods?

Almost all feeling of discontent comes from doing work you really don't want to do and from being in relationships you don't really want to be in. It's that TRAPPED-IN-A-CAGE feeling. You wish you were somewhere else but you have no idea how to get from POINT A to POINT B. You begin to reason with yourself that you have no choice. You convince yourself you have to work a job you hate because you have bills to pay. You stay in bad relationships because you don't want to rock the boat.

To be flexible means to start listening. You take a left turn on what seemed like a straight road (to nowhere). You allow yourself to be led in new directions.

This can be scary, especially for us "control freaks!"

Most addicts think things are supposed to be done in a certain way.

We like to know in advance what's going to happen next! We like to know where the road leads! We want to know the beginning, middle and end. No surprises, please!

I went along this self-appointed path until finally I was so bored out of my mind that I was willing to start taking a few risks. I allowed myself to be open to the Holy Spirit and His Plan. Then life started to get fun again, a thrilling adventure full of magnificent possibilities.

Becoming flexible is characterized by having the willingness to try new things, to experiment, to bend your rules, and to go with the flow.

You stop trying to swim upstream. The river current is hard and fast, and it's a waste of energy trying to struggle against the current. It's time to go with the flow. You start to relax and let yourself flow downstream, naturally and peacefully. You stop kicking. You stop striving. You stop thrashing. You turn from your front side to your back side, and you start to float. It's wonderful!

Being flexible is easy when your priorities are in order.

My first priority is that my life belongs to God. I go wherever He wants me to go. That's my #1 priority. That's the whole game plan. My life belongs to God. Period. This means that anything can happen next.

Right now I run a Bed & Breakfast in Wisconsin, but my life belongs to God. It's very possible I could lose this house and this job this afternoon. That's okay. I am open to the possibility of something brand new occurring. I want to go wherever the Holy Spirit needs me to go. I trust in God. I hang on to nothing. I let Him lead the way. This is true flexibility.

My life is the canvas. The Holy Spirit is the artist. Pure creativity. The picture is constantly changing.

I am being flexible with food nowadays. I am experimenting. I am letting things flow naturally. I had a hard-fast rule about life being too short, so eat dessert first. LOL. I stuck with this rule, come hell or high water! If I was hungry, I ate sugar first. It was my right! Give me freedom! Or give me death! I defend my right to eat cake! LOL. But now I'm being more flexible. In my defenselessness, my safety lies. I am staying open to new instruction. What feels good? Am I clinging to a past idea? Or does the Holy Spirit want me to turn down a new road?

This week I started getting a very strong inclination to start juicing. At first I was totally pissed off because I don't want to eat healthy! And after all, I thought I wasn't dieting here, right?? Don't make me start juicing when I prefer pancakes with maple syrup for lunch! LOL. I realized I wasn't being very flexible. I was fighting against the current. I laughed right out loud. I'm laughing at myself a lot nowadays. So I got out the juicer and I bought a big bag of carrots, celery and apples. I'm letting myself be led down this road. *It feels good*, which is a marvelous surprise!

I am willing to yield. I'm listening.

I am responsive to change.

Exercise #1:

Change your plans if they don't feel right. Start listening. Be flexible, willing to yield, responsive to change.

And remember also: JOY IS THE BAROMETER.

Whenever you are not entirely joyful about your plans, then something has gone wrong. When you are following the Holy Spirit's plans, you will be excited like a little kid. Work feels like play. Meeting friends is exciting. You'll be happy like a teenager in the first flush of love. Everything feels effortless and easy. If this is not the case, then you're following your own plan. STOP. If life feels like a struggle to you, then you are swimming upstream, fighting against the current. STOP.

Just stop.

Stop fighting the current. Stop struggling. Stop trying to keep your head above water. You might think you will drown, but instead you'll start floating. Just try it!

Day 26

Dealing with limitations

When Marielle suggested "Dealing with limitations" as a possible topic for this 40-day course, I shot it down immediately.

I said "There is no such thing as limitations, only excuses."

Marielle was silent so I said to her: "Okay, name me some limitations."

She said: "no money, not good enough, not enough time, too old, too young."

Oh. Okay. I see what we are talking about here. All those things are excuses, but I guess you're right: most people call them limitations. DEALING WITH LIMITATIONS.

Limitations are excuses that you have interposed between you and the life you really want to live. Limitations are blocks and obstacles that stall you and keep you, well, limited!

They are called LIMIT-ATIONS because they limit you. They keep you confined to a small space.

A limit is a boundary. It's a fence to keep you in.

A limit is a restriction.

A limit is a lack of capacity, a handicap, restrictive weakness, an inability to think creatively.

But let's be honest: Do you really have limitations? What are they?

I have a physical disability. Deafness. I have never considered it a disability or limitation. It's been a blessing in disguise in many ways. It forced me to be more focused. By necessity, I had to learn to listen closely and pay attention to what people were saying to me or I missed it entirely. I literally cannot focus on two things at once. I cannot talk with music playing in the background. It's impossible for me. When this is happening, I neither hear the talking nor the music, just noise that all blends together.

So I have had to learn to "deal with limitations."

One thing I have learned is that there is not a single limitation in all the world that can stop you from achieving your goal if you are determined and focused.

The theme of this week is CREATIVITY and dealing with limitations is about being creative. You come up with solutions that work with whatever limitations you are facing. No money to live the life you want? You'll find a way. No time to pursue your goal? You'll find a way.

If you really want something, you'll find a way.

I've been deaf since the 3rd grade, but I wanted to do well in school. So I found a way. I sat in the front row of the classroom. I studied with increased dedication and the result is that I was an A student. Most people are surprised to find out I'm deaf (unless you are really close friends with me, and then it's obvious).

One of the big limitations people come up with is "no support." They think they cannot do what they want to do because there is no one around cheering them on, inspiring them, coaching them, or encouraging them. People think they could achieve more if their environment was more conducive to their goals; more quiet and supportive.

Take eating healthy for example. Many will use the excuse/limitation that they can't eat healthy because their family wants to eat big meals and junk food.

It's based on fear of ridicule and fear that you'll be abandoned.

It's the "What Will the Neighbors Think" syndrome.

Or maybe you think you can't be an artist because you have kids, a job, and a husband that's not interested in your work.

I thought I couldn't publish a book because I didn't have any money and I couldn't get a publisher or agent interested in my work. At the time, I thought I was all alone. Poor Lisa! I thought everyone else had all the talent and good luck. I thought "if only I had money, I could do so much more! Then I could publish a book! If only I had a team of people working with me, then I could start being really creative and productive! Then I could make a difference in the world! Then I could do work I love. I could hire an editor. I could hire a marketing team. I could hire graphic art designers. But no. Poor Lisa. I have no money. I can't do anything. No one cares. I'm all alone. I'm doomed to a life of mediocrity and part-time minimum wage jobs that I can't stand."

Excuses. Excuses. Excuses.

So what did I do? I started a Wordpress blog for free. I started writing on a daily basis. I wanted to be a published writer but I wasn't writing every day. I was spending the mass majority of my day in fantasy land thinking about how awesome it would be to be a published author. Meanwhile I wasn't writing! haha. I'm laughing now. At the time it wasn't so funny. But now it's hilarious. The life I wanted to live was always there for me and all I had to do was get a little creative, and claim it for myself. FOR FREE!

I started supporting and encouraging myself. I let go of my ideas about how reaching my goal was supposed to look.

Speaking of her own experience, Marielle once said, "I learned to do what was necessary; to take baby steps and only look at THE ACTION needed to handle what was directly in front of me. I let go of the result."

GREAT ADVICE!

Take baby steps.
Do what is necessary.
Look at the action needed to handle only what is directly in front of you.
Let go of the result.

GREAT FUN EXERCISE #1!

Write a list of what you would do, be, have, buy if you had all the money and all the time in the world.

Exercise #2 (even more fun than Exercise #1!):

Step into the fear. Do what scares you.

There is never, ever, NEVER going to be a moment when there is no fear. Never. The moment you are waiting for will never arrive. The timing is never right. Again, I repeat: THE TIMING IS NEVER RIGHT. There is always going to be fear. So step right into it. Do what scares you. Do something terrifying.

There is only today. There are always going to be limits. You are never going to have all your ducks lined up in a row. There is never enough money and never enough time, but that is no excuse. Start moving in the direction of where you want to go. Determine what you want and head in that direction.

Day 27

Vacationing

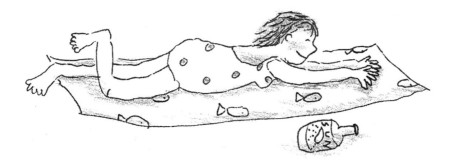

What is your perfect idea of a vacation?

When was the last time you took a vacation?

Vacationing is about finding A SWEET LITTLE SPOT.

Vacationing is about indulging. It is about luxury, relaxation, and the creation of new and happy memories.

Vacationing is a break from rules, diets and rigid structure.

The perfect vacation for me is where there is nothing to do; no plans, no worries, and no cares.

My perfect vacation includes sun, water, wind, and lots of lounging around. I love mornings, and the perfect vacation to me is waking up leisurely without an alarm clock and then lounging around in a bathrobe, drinking coffee, reading, writing, with all the windows and doors open so I can feel the wind and water.

I like the simplicity of meals on vacation. I like eating in restaurants to taste local cuisine. I love cooking together with family. I love room-service. I love outside cafes with a friend.

My ideal vacations have no agenda. I like to lounge on beaches and porches with a book. If there is any traveling involved in my ideal vacation it is only to get to a beach, porch or restaurant where there is more lounging, eating, cappuccinos, and reading.

Paradise!

Exercise #1:

What constitutes your ideal vacation?

For some people, it involves traveling, sight-seeing and being active. For others, the perfect vacation is about relaxing. Visualize your perfect vacation. What do your days look like on vacation?

Exercise #2:

Plan a vacation.

The anticipation and planning is one of the best parts of vacationing. It gives you time to get excited.

Think about where you want to go and what you want to do.

Plan a daily vacation (a break in your day - it could be ten minutes to an hour). This would include taking walks, going to a cafe with a friend, writing letters, sending postcards, walking barefoot in the grass, sitting in the sun, going to a spa, getting a manicure, swimming in a pool, eating a meal prepared by someone else, having breakfast in bed, sleeping in, etc.

Plan a dream vacation. Where have you always wanted to go? Start planning. Start saving. Buy travel books. Where do you want to go?

Exercise #3:

Take a day off every week.

Most people don't take days off anymore. I'm like most people and my week is packed with activities. But in the name of my own healing, I need to take a day for myself. I choose Tuesdays. It's a play day. It's vacation time. Friday, Saturday, and Sunday I am busy with the Bed & Breakfast. Mondays and Wednesday I have a radio show. Tuesday is a great day for me to relax after a busy weekend of guests, laundry, cleaning rooms and cooking.

Taking a vacation is about adding PLAY into your life.

Vacationing is a spatial reference. It's a sweet spot.

Marielle calls it "a fairy spot." It's a place where you are out of this world, away from all seriousness and problems. It's a place where you are nourished and happy.

Instead of comfort foods, find comfort time, and find comfort space.

Day 28
Superstar!

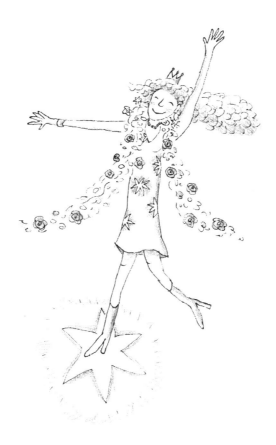

You are the light of the world!

You are the brightest star in the whole universe. Your name is written in the stars.

"Look up and see His Word among the stars, where He has set your Name along with His. Look up and find your certain destiny the world would hide but God would have you see."
                    ACIM, Epilogue

"The Thought God holds of you is like a star, unchangeable in an eternal sky. So high in Heaven is it set that those outside of Heaven know not it is there. But still and white and lovely will it shine through all eternity. There was no time it was not there; no instant when its light grew dimmer or less perfect ever was. Who knows the Father knows this light, for He is the eternal sky which holds it safe, forever lifted up and anchored sure. Its perfect purity does not depend on whether it is seen on earth or not. The sky embraces it, and softly holds it in its perfect place, which is as far from earth as earth from Heaven. It is not the distance nor the time which keeps this star invisible to earth. But those who seek for idols cannot know this star is there."

Urtext, Chapter 30, Beyond All Idols

You are a Super Star!
Bright Shining Star.
Pure Light.
You are the light of the world.

Today's topic is about shining bright, being the SUPER STAR that you are.

You are the center of the universe. You are the brightest thing this world has ever seen.
Does your life reflect this fact?
Does your appearance reflect this truth?
You are a star!

Many people "hide their light under a bushel." They are afraid to "sparkle, shimmer and shine."

Be aware of the first step into hell because the rest of the steps come quickly.

"Brothers, take not one step in the descent to hell. For, having taken one, you will not recognize the rest for what they are. And they WILL follow. Attack in any form has placed your foot upon the twisted stairway that leads from Heaven... How can you know whether you chose the stairs to Heaven or the way to hell? Quite easily. How do you feel?"

ACIM, Chapter 23, The Laws of Chaos

I never noticed I was moving into sloth when I started wearing baggy sweatpants around the house. They were more comfortable. Then I stopped taking a morning shower or getting dressed until around noon. I was doing all my writing and working in my bathrobe. I didn't comb my hair. Instead I threw it up in a bun in an elastic band. It all started innocently enough, right? With the oversized sweatpants, I felt like I could eat more. With no one around, I got lazy. It's no surprise I gained 50 pounds in a year. I was shocked when I stepped on the scale. 50 pounds!?! What?? I actually thought the battery in the scale wasn't working and I went to the store and bought a new one. LOL. The battery was working fine. I didn't see the weight gain while it was occurring because I was not paying attention.

Super Stardom changed all that.

Super Stardom gives you purpose, direction and clarity.

Super Star! makes you start caring about your life and your self.

I started thinking that I was like Jim Carrey in the movie *The Truman Show* and that the whole universe was watching my every move. I began to think that the cameras were running constantly in my life, aimed at me. Being the lead actress in my own life kept me on my toes.

With the camera rolling, I began making my bed in the morning. I started taking showers again, first thing. I threw out all my clothes that were tattered and torn. These clothes were unacceptable to donate to charity and yet I was wearing them. This should have told me something!

The name of this 40-day program is *IT MATTERS TOTALLY.*

You matter totally. Your life matters totally. You are a Super Star!

Exercise #1:

Find a way to be extravagant and bright.

My bible is *The Bombshell Manual of Style* by Laren Stover. It sits on my nightstand and I know many sentences by heart because I have incorporated the lessons into my daily life. I've morphed myself into a Brunette Bombshell by sheer decision. I was not born a Bombshell (not by any stretch of the imagination), but I decided I wanted to become one and that became my goal. Being a Bombshell seemed like a fun way to go through life.

Here are some beautiful one-liners from Laren Stover's book *The Bombshell Manual of Style*:

The Bombshell is authentic.
The Bombshell is vulnerable.
The Bombshell radiates confidence.
The Bombshell puts glamour before comfort.
The Bombshell laughs, leans, listens, looks and touches.
The Bombshell is comfortable and familiar with her body.
The Bombshell expresses her feelings as openly as she displays her curves.

Fun stuff.

A Course in Miracles says: " We pause but for a moment more, to play our final, happy game upon this earth."
    ACIM, Lesson 153, In my defenselessness my safety lies

You should be having fun.

Joy is the barometer.

Exercise #2:

Dress up. Be aware of your appearance.

Most addicts simply do not care about themselves or their appearance. They start to slide into sloth, usually without even realizing it. They begin to give excuses that they prefer to be comfortable. This is the result of a lazy mind. Be careful!

You are designed to shine!!

WEEK 5
RECEIVING

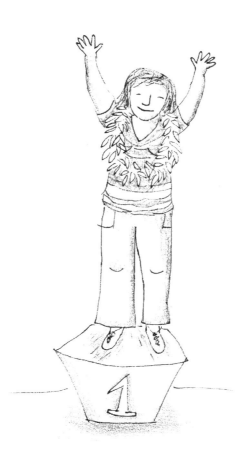

Day 29

Consistency

The theme of this new week, Week 5, is RECEIVING.

The topic on our first day on the theme of Receiving is CONSISTENCY.

In the original manuscript of *A Course in Miracles* (which is called the Urtext), Chapter 7 is titled "The Consistency of the Kingdom." In the published version, they changed the word "Consistency" to "Gifts." I have no idea why they did that, but consistency is the word meant to be there. I like the phrase "The Consistency of the Kingdom." That makes sense to me. In Heaven, everything is the same. It's consistent! There is only love! There are no highs and lows.

Is your life consistent?
Are you consistent?

Most people alternate between happy and sad, high and low, and up and down. They go back and forth between certainty and uncertainty. The only consistent thing in most people is inconsistency!

In God, there is consistency. He gives only love. He doesn't change His mood based on the weather.

In God, everything is equal. Giving and receiving are the same. There are no differences.

Most food addicts are on the giving side, being overly generous because they really, REALLY want to receive. They give to get. Most are not even consciously aware of this kind of behavior. They think the only way to receive is to give, give, give, give, give. They over-extend. If you are giving to get, you are giving nothing. Giving to get is attack. Most food addicts cannot imagine that someone will give them a gift without their doing something nice first. But this is all wrong. This is false learning.

You are totally lovable! You are given gifts all day long, from start to finish. Are you noticing them? They come in many forms, through many different sources, and through many people, quite often from strangers.

The universe is constantly giving you gifts, but are you consistently receiving? Are your eyes open to see all that is being given to you? Are you consistently appreciative of all the gifts that are given to you on a daily basis?

You are being given gifts every minute of the day, but are you receiving them? Do you notice all the kindness around you? Have you accepted your gifts? They are right there in front of you. Look at them and take them for your own.

"Your Guest (the Christ) HAS come. You asked Him, and He came. You did not hear Him enter, for you did not wholly welcome Him. And yet His gifts came with Him. He has laid them at your feet, and asks you now that you will look on them, and take them for your own. He NEEDS your help in giving them to all who walk apart, believing they are separate and alone. They WILL be healed when you accept your gifts, because your Guest will welcome everyone whose feet have touched the holy ground whereon you stand, and where His gifts for them are laid. You do not see how much you now can GIVE, because of everything you have received."
Urtext, Chapter 29, The Coming of the Guest

Here is a FACT: You cannot give truly until you have received. So, today's lesson is about opening yourself up to receive consistently.

This week's theme is about receiving. First you receive, and then you can give. This requires a determination to be consistent, because probably your first reaction in every situation is to give. But now you are learning to receive. You are learning that to receive is what giving is! Giving and receiving are the same.

Here is what Jesus tells us in *A Course in Miracles*:

"God's laws are always fair, and PERFECTLY consistent. By giving, you receive. But to receive is to accept, NOT to get. It is impossible not to have, but it is possible NOT TO KNOW YOU HAVE. The recognition of HAVING is the willingness for giving, and only by this willingness, can you RECOGNIZE what you have. What you give is therefore the value you put on what you have, being the exact measure of the value you PUT upon it. And this, in turn, is the measure of HOW MUCH YOU WANT IT."
Urtext, Chapter 8, The Answer to Prayer

Amazing, huh? You're receiving all the time but you probably neither notice nor appreciate it because you set the value low.

When you "give to get" you have already determined ahead of time what you want to receive. And it almost never comes in the form you have demanded, so you are blind to all the other gifts that come your way.

Such is the human condition.

This 40-day course is about opening your eyes to the gifts that are all around you.

CONSISTENCY.

Receiving is often difficult for an addict. First, you don't believe you deserve to be loved or given a gift, and then you automatically think you have to give back. What an interesting predicament!

You want to receive (love, appreciation, affection, gifts, flowers, words of praise) but then you immediately feel guilty when someone gives to you!

What an insane place to be!

When people gave to me it made me feel badly. It made me feel inferior in some way. I didn't feel I deserved gifts. To me everything was a scoreboard!

If someone gave to me, I thought it meant I had to give back!

OH NO! THE BALL IS IN MY COURT! I GOTTA SWING IT BACK INTO THEIR COURT!

And not only that, I thought my "thank-you-for-giving-me-a-gift gesture" had to be better than the gift that was given to me. The whole thing was an exhausting game.

I was so used to "giving to get" that I automatically assumed that everyone else was a subtle manipulator like myself. Receiving made me suspicious and anxious. It made me feel like someone was trying to get something from me.

If someone gave me flowers, it meant they wanted sex.

If someone gave me a compliment, it meant they were preparing to ask me for a huge favor.

If someone praised my cooking, I immediately thought they were dropping a hint to cook them three meals a day.

I was suspicious of everyone and everything.

I never received/enjoyed a single gift even though gifts were being given to me on a daily basis. I was incapable of receiving. I was too busy wondering what someone's ulterior motive was! I never allowed myself to luxuriate in a gift because my mind was already racing ahead about how I could give back.

It was like an exhausting tennis match!

It was easier for me if people just didn't give to me at all.

But this blocks the flow of God's Love. This is a major obstruction in the river of life. When you block your ability to receive eventually everything else starts to go wrong.

Exercise #1:

Stop giving. Learn to say "no" when people ask you to give.

This might sound like a strange thing to say, but you need to practice this idea because most addicts have no idea what giving is. The automatic response for most addicts is "Yes, okay" with the automatic built-in thought that they'll get something out of it.

Addicts say "yes" because they feel guilty or because they are being selfish (wanting to boost their image, trying to get something out of the deal, or to rack up "brownie points"). This is because all addicts know they'll need something later, and if they say "no" to a request for help, they won't get help when they need it.

These are all false ideas.

Most giving is not genuine giving (in the true sense of the word) so we want you to stop it. Stop giving. Start saying "no" when people ask you to give. Stop trying to figure out how you can be nice to someone. Stop.

Most giving is subtle manipulation in disguise.

So we want you to stop it. Stop trying to be nice all the time. Stop trying to figure out how to please or help your brother.

It's impossible to give without receiving.

So give to yourself and see how much you receive.

Exercise #2:

Open yourself to receive.

God longs to give you everything. Your brother longs to give you everything. The whole universe wants to shower you with gifts. You need to open yourself up to receive all that is waiting for you.

Exercise #3:

Be consistent.

Pick an area of your life where you can begin to be consistent. It can either be an eternal theme (consistently happy, consistently taking care of yourself, being vigilant for God and His Kingdom) or it can be a theme encompassing an area of time and space (completing a project, showing up every day to do the exercises in this program, completing the workbook lessons of *A Course in Miracles* in 365 days, honoring your word, drinking *x* number of glasses of water a day, working out *x* number of minutes every day, etc.)

Day 30

Connecting

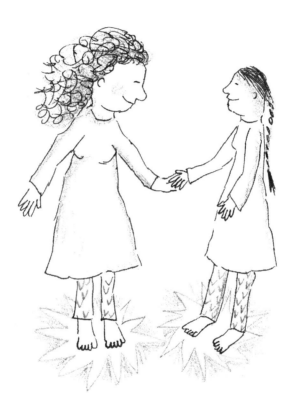

Most spiritual seekers and addicts have one thing in common: ESCAPISM.

Addicts try to escape from their bodies and from their lives. They escape into food, books, alcohol, sex, other people's problems and busyness. All such attempts are made in order to avoid looking at *themselves*. They detach from other people. They prefer to be alone to live in fantasies about the past or the future. They attach to other people. They prefer to look at other people's lives instead of their own.

Rather than be squarely in the moment, fully alive within the body, they live in their minds in a manner that is really outside of themselves, and not connected.

Addicts have a lot of creative energy and unfortunately they waste it on fantasy.

Connecting is about claiming your own energy. It is about being in your body, being present in your relationships, showing up fully in your work, and living your life today. Now.

Forget about how great your life will be in the future when you are healed of food addiction.

HOW DO YOU FEEL RIGHT NOW?

Connect with your body.

Connect with this moment.

Your body is constantly sending you signals – it's hungry, it's thirsty, it needs rest, it needs fresh air, it needs quiet time - and by the time sickness shows up in you, you have been receiving signals for a long time and ignoring them.

Most people get sick because they need to relax and be nurtured. They can't possibly fathom that they could take a holiday/vacation to rest and play for a few days (weeks, months or years) without being totally sick.

Years ago I stopped working for other people. I saw the importance of living every day authentically. It took courage to quit my job without a safety net but I figured this was smarter than getting cancer.

I wanted to spend my days at home in great health and action. My friends and family thought I was crazy. They wanted an explanation. They said "you can't just quit your job! You can't just stay home all day! How are you going to pay your bills??"

Hell if I knew, but I needed to do this.

If people get a serious illness they have a great excuse to stay at home and have other people take care of them.

I decided to bypass that route. I didn't need an excuse. I didn't need sickness. I simply made a decision that from that day on I was working for myself at home as a writer, and that was the end of the story.

Connecting to the present moment requires BRUTAL HONESTY and THE ABILITY TO STOP EXPLAINING YOURSELF.

The reason people feel a constant need to talk, talk, talk, talk, talk is because of their own guilt. They feel like they have to explain themselves if they are not being productive. The guilt is so overwhelming that they need to get rid of it by dumping it on their brother. Please don't do this anymore. Your brother doesn't need your guilt. He doesn't need an explanation.

But YOU need to feel the emotion and connect with the energy totally, rather than try to remove it, or project it from yourself.

Here's what Jesus tells us:

"The ultimate purpose of projection, as the ego uses it, is ALWAYS to get rid of guilt... For much as the ego wants to RETAIN guilt, YOU find it intolerable. For guilt stands in the way of your remembering God, Whose pull is so strong that YOU cannot resist it. On this issue, then, the deepest split of all occurs, for if you are to RETAIN guilt, as the ego insists, YOU CANNOT BE YOU. Only by persuading you that IT is you, could the ego possibly induce you to PROJECT guilt, and thereby keep it in your mind.

You PROJECT guilt to get rid of it, but you actually merely CONCEAL it. You DO experience guilt FEELINGS, but you have NO IDEA OF WHY. On the contrary, you associate them with a weird assortment of EGO ideals, which the ego claims you have failed. But you have no idea that you are failing the Son of God, by seeing HIM as guilty.

Believing you are no longer YOU, you do not realize that you are failing YOURSELF."

Urtext, Chapter 12, The Problem of Guilt

This is very important that you see this. As long as you talk to other people, you start to feel better. But it's only a temporary band-aid. It feels good to get rid of your guilt and relieve some of your burden. This always makes you feel better, doesn't it? But then what happens? You start to feel bad again.

The reason is because you never deal with the guilt. You never go into the pain. You never heal the core issue. Instead you attempt to share the pain and guilt by giving it away. This will never work. You need to connect with the discomfort and let it heal. You need to be brutally honest.

You need to be in your body. You need to be connected to the present moment.

Be one with it.

Exercise #1

Be brutally honest.

Feel what you feel. Connect with yourself. Do you feel jealous, not appreciated, angry, bored, or hungry? Feel it. Be in your body. Connect with the energy. Be in the moment. Be in the emotion. FEEL IT.

Most addicts have developed a skill of numbing themselves to the point that they can't feel anything.

Exercise #2:

Stop explaining yourself.

Feel what you feel without constant commentary to everyone in your life. There is no need to express everything that happens to you. What you feel is no one else's business.

Exercise #3:

Be aware when you are connected.

Connect with your body.
Connect with others.
Connect with God.
Connect with this moment.
Connect with your children.
Connect with your computer.
Connect with your pets.
Connect with the food you are eating.

Be one with everything.

Have you ever been talking with someone and you suddenly realize they're not listening? There is no connection. It's like a telephone call that suddenly has bad reception or no dial tone. The mass majority of people are blind to this. They keep talking. They keep sharing. But no one is listening. These two individuals are "out of range" from out of range. You don't need to fix this. Just be aware when you lose the connection.

Connecting is directly related to receiving. When you are connected (with another, with your work, with the moment) you begin to feel the power of God, and *there* is your inheritance. *There* is where the miracle lies.

A Course in Miracles, Lesson 77:

I am entitled to miracles.

"You will RECEIVE miracles because of what God is. And you will offer miracles because you are one with God. Again, how simple is salvation!"

Connect, love yourself, and step into the true miracle of you!

Day 31

Balance

My addictive behavior can be summed up in three words: ALL OR NOTHING.

I was the Queen of Extremes.

My whole life I rarely did anything on middle ground. I lived on opposite poles on the scale. The pendulum swung from deprivation to excess.

I was either living on 800 calories a day OR 3000 calories a day. The word "moderation" simply did not exist in my vocabulary.

Balance? What's that? I have no idea what you're talking about.

In my world everything had to be black or white. Either I was fasting/dieting with lots of restrictions or my life was an all-you-can-eat-buffet with no rules.

This 40-day program has calmed me down. It has helped CENTER me. Balance is about living life in the center. When you are balanced, you are not tipping the scale on either side. You are right in the middle. You are neither high nor low.

BALANCE IS ABOUT BEING CENTERED.

What I've learned is that trying to hold myself to an extreme ideal is not natural. Quite literally, I was out of balance. I was off kilter. At times I was too light and flighty, practically ready to fly away if someone looked at me the wrong way or said an unkind word. And all other times I was too heavy in the world, too serious, not flowing. But never in balance.

Balance is harmony.

Balance in a stereo is where both speakers produce the same average sound level. One speaker is not drowning the other out.

Physical balance is a state of equilibrium, an equal distribution of weight.

In wine, balance is the degree to which all attributes are in harmony, with none either too prominent or deficient.

BALANCE.

I know for myself, my addiction threw me all out of whack, with none of my attributes in harmony. I was always either way too loud or way too quiet. I was too pushy or too meek. I swung between extroverted and introverted. There was no middle ground. I was continuously trying to control my behavior. I was always attempting to figure out how I should "be." Should I be more showy? Should I be more quiet? Should I stand out more? Should I step back? Should I be more aggressive? Should I be more gentle?

I was constantly attempting to control my behavior, which disrupted the natural flow of things.

Nature is sometimes calm and sometimes full of fury. She is both sunny and stormy. But nature balances herself. In times of *extreme* weather when nature is out of balance (as is happening lately with pollution caused by excess human consumption) you see chaos, destruction, floods and tornadoes. Nothing is in harmony.

So it is with food addiction. Nothing is in harmony.

When you go to any extreme, it throws off the natural balance.

Whenever I would decide to go on a diet, I would make a huge sweeping loud declaration and tell everyone I knew:

"I'm fasting!"
"I'm not eating sugar anymore!"
"I'm doing a raw diet, eating only fruits, nuts and vegetables!"
"Look at me!"

In a balanced state, my mind is calm. I'm happy. I eat when I'm hungry. I don't tell the world over a loudspeaker about every calorie I'm consuming (or not consuming). In a balanced state, I'm creative and active.

In an extreme state, all I can do is think about food. In an extreme state, I'm cranky, bored, tired, obsessed and fearful. It's like being a fish out of water. In an extreme state, I'm not in my natural environment and I suffer because of it.

Exercise #1:

Practice living in balance.

See where your life is out of balance. Do you spend all your time indoors? Then start spending a few hours outside. Take your work to the beach. Take your cell phone outside and sit in the sun.

Do you eat only one kind of food? All carbs? All protein? All sugar? Try balancing it out. Start experimenting with food. Strive for balance in your meals.

Exercise #2:

Check in with your body.

Are you sick or healthy?
Do you have back pain?
Headaches?
Is your neck stiff?
Do you breathe normally?
How flexible are you?

When you are out of balance, your body will send you signals.

If you are holding yourself in an extreme condition (too much or too little of something), your body is probably rigid and tense.

Exercise #3:

Balance work/family/play.

Try to balance your day with work, family and play.

How much time each day do you spend working?
Playing?
Spending time with loved ones?

Look at the ratio and see where you are out of balance. Find ways to balance your life.

Exercise #4:

Do one thing at a time.

The addict is classically trying to do five things all at once. Right now I need to finish writing this article, the lawn needs watering, I need to clean some B & B rooms for guests coming in today, I want to walk the dogs, I need to eat lunch, go to the grocery store, and create an audio with Marielle. All these things are clamoring for my attention right now. Finding balance is to do one thing at a time, and to do it well. Complete one project and move to the next.

Balance is about staying focused. It is about getting priorities straight and doing what needs to be done, without trying to do everything at once.

Addicts are famous for overwhelming themselves with too many projects.

Today, practice balance. Make time for yourself. Make time for work. Make time for play. Make time for family. Balance.

Day 32

Strengthening your core

Everything in time and space is designed to distract you from remembering you are the light of the world. That's neither good nor bad, but the question is: "How long does it take you to get back to your center, to find your core again?"

Did you know that all airplanes are off-course 99% of the time as they travel to their destination? The pilot's job is to continually bring the plane back on track until it arrives at its destination.

Do you think pilots beat themselves up that their airplanes are off course 99% of the time? No. That's just how it is. It's a known fact that a plane will be off-course almost the entire flight. A pilot's job is to stay alert and get the plane back on track. A pilot is in a state of constant correction.

You are a pilot, your body is the vehicle, and your job is to stay alert and keep constantly correcting when you go off track.

Hopefully this analogy will help you next time you fly off track in rage, jealousy, or depression. These emotions are neither good nor bad. HOWEVER, how far off course do you allow yourself to go?

Do you stay angry for an hour, a day, or a week?
If a friend upsets you, how long does it take for you to get back to your center where you are peaceful, happy and calm?

Strengthening your core.

Bring yourself back to the place where you are happy and inspired again.

I find it interesting that when people make mistakes, they keep going down that path until they are 700 miles off course. The best thing to do if you have lost your peace of mind is to STOP, then bring yourself back to your core.

If you have a "bad" eating day, do you beat yourself up while continuing to follow a path of self-sabotage (going 700 miles off course) or do you get back on track?

Exercise #1:

FIND YOUR CENTER.

What is your core?

It's impossible to bring yourself back to your core (to align yourself with your center) if you do not know what your core is.

It could be light, joy, creativity, strength, nurturing, certainty, love, beauty, calm, peace.

Your center could also be your stomach or your solar plexus. This is a good technique when you start allowing yourself to be pulled into other people's dramas. Just focus on your stomach and bring your energy back to yourself.

Be alert.
Realize when you are off center.
Get back on track.

Exercise #2:

KNOW YOUR DESTINATION.

Where are you headed?

In order to fly a plane from Point A to Point B, you need to know where you are going. What is your goal?

If your goal is happiness, are you heading in that direction?

How far off the mark do you allow yourself to go before bringing your thoughts back to remembering the path you have set yourself upon.

Exercise #3:

Create an emergency nurturing package.

This could be a toy box filled with dolls, games, magazines and treasures; a hope chest with favorite photo albums and art supplies; a bookcase filled with books that make you happy; a box filled with stationery and pens; a cabinet in your bathroom with all your favorite spa products; a glass jar filled with money for a "rainy day", etc.

Exercise #4:

Create an emergency phrase that you can use at all times to calm yourself down.

I use the phrase "Gorgeous for God." This helps me remember my ultimate purpose.

Some more good phrases are:
"Focus!"
"Center, Center, Center."
"Breathe."

Or you can use some of the phrases Jesus has given you in *A Course in Miracles:*

> "I am the light of the world."
> "God's Will for me is perfect happiness."
> "I am here *only* to be truly helpful."

Day 33

The wisdom of YOUR body

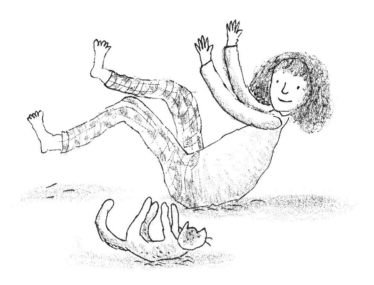

Food addicts are probably the most knowledgeable individuals on the planet when it comes to THE body. They know about weight loss methods, body functions, calorie/protein requirements, exercise techniques, yoga, alternative therapies, healing remedies, drug information, ayurveda, vitamins and supplements. They are experts in the field of health. They know what is good and bad for the body. They could practically be medical doctors or pharmacists.

Addicts know everything there is to know about the body: illness, wellness, and health - and yet many are sick. Why is this?

The reason is they don't know about the wisdom of THEIR body. They know about THE body, but not their own body.

The wisdom of YOUR body is about learning to listen to what YOU need to take care of yourself. Your body knows what it needs to eat. It knows how much exercise and rest it needs. Forget about rules of nutrition. Forget about all the books and articles you've read. Forget about what has been successful for other people.

Today's topic is about tuning into YOUR body and watching for signals and listening to what it is saying to you.

Your body is giving signals all day long. Are you paying attention? Think of a car. It needs gas and oil to run at optimal performance. You need to take care of your car if you expect it to run well. You watch for signals. You listen for funny noises. No one in their right mind would let a gas tank go to empty and then say: "Oh, it will be fine. I don't need to do anything. It's fine. No worries."

No, it's not fine. It will die on the side of the road without gas. If you don't put oil in a car, it destroys the engine. If you don't take care of it, it will eventually break down.

And so it is with your body. You must start paying attention to it. Are you running on an empty tank of gas? Are you taking care of yourself?

Exercise #1:

Be your own specialist.

Exercise #2:

Be your own nutritionist.

Exercise #3:

Be your own personal trainer when it comes to exercise.

Addicts are great at giving advice. They know what is good for other people, but are not so great when it comes to themselves.

Remember, *your body is giving signals all day long.*

What do you need?

What would be some simple practical ways for you to take care of yourself so that you are operating at optimal levels?

Your body is sending you signals. What are the signals you are receiving?

Exercise #4:

Start checking in with your body on a daily basis.

Tune in. Pay attention. What are some of the signals you are receiving? Are you tired? Having heartburn? Stomach acid? Muscle aches? Back pain? Goosebumps? Feeling hot or cold? Experiencing blockage? Lethargy? Irregular heart beat? Difficulty in breathing?

Remember, your body is sending you signals all the time. It's like a car. You begin to "feel" when something is not quite right. It's easier to take preventive care (bringing it in for tune-ups and oil changes) rather than wait until the engine blows up.

And so it is with you. The practice is to take care of yourself – drink lots of water, get lots of rest, play, eat great meals, laugh – and you won't have any problems. If you do start to "feel" something is not right with you, then catch these signals as soon as you notice them and begin a program of extreme self-care before these signals become a full-blown disease.

Your body knows exactly what it needs. It is wise and full of wisdom. It knows exactly how to take care of itself. Your job is to listen, watch for signals, and then follow instructions. If the gas tank says empty and a red warning light is flashing, please pay attention and do something. Don't ignore the signals you are receiving. Your body is wise. It's trying to help you.

Day 34

Listening

Listening is a skill that involves all of your senses, not just your ears.

Most people think that listening has to do with words, language, sound and voices; but real hearing is about sensing, sensation, gut feeling and intuition. Listening can sometimes involve words and sound, but often listening comes in the form of a feeling.

To listen is to pay attention.

True listening involves waiting, relaxing and being in stillness. *A Course in Miracles* is uncompromising. It says there are two voices within you speaking. One Voice is the Holy Spirit and the other voice is the ego.

When you listen to the Holy Spirit, you will always feel calm and happy.

When you listen to the voice of the ego, you will feel agitated, depressed, confused, angry, nervous and tired.

The same goes for what other people are saying to you. If you listen to someone and you start to feel badly, that's the voice of the ego. If you start to feel happy, that's the Holy Spirit. The Holy Spirit will never lead you into fear or confusion.

If you are being led into fear or confusion, listen!

The topic of listening is about TAKING YOUR TEMPERATURE about what you are saying to yourself and what others are saying to you. HOW DO YOU FEEL?

Do you feel happy, anxious, guilty or joyful with the thoughts you are thinking about yourself?? Do other people's words make you feel inspired, tired, upset or confused? When listening to someone talk, do you feel tense or relaxed? When sitting quietly with yourself, how do you feel?

Believe it or not, becoming aware of your body's signals is an exercise in LISTENING.

Do you feel rushed, bored, overwhelmed, or sick? Then you are listening to the voice of the e-GO.

Go, Go, Go. Rush, Rush, Rush. This voice leads you straight into hell (and probably straight to the fridge.)

Do you feel excited, happy, playful and inspired? That's the Holy Spirit.

Joy is the barometer.

The most important thing you can do for yourself is to find a thought that feels good, and to do things that make you feel happy.

Joy is the barometer.

Are you listening to the way you feel? Are you listening to the thoughts in your head? What do you hear? The Holy Spirit is speaking to you all the time, all day long, telling you exactly what to do, where to go, and what to say. Listening to His Voice and following His instruction will bring you into an experience of constant joy.

"The Holy Spirit's Voice is as loud as your willingness to listen."
ACIM, Chapter 8, The Body as Means or End

"Listen to MY Voice, Learn to undo the error, and DO something to correct it. The first two are not enough. The real members of MY party are ACTIVE workers. The power to work Miracles BELONGS to you. I will create the right opportunities for you to do them. But you must be ready and willing to do them, since you are already able to. Doing them will bring conviction in the ability. I repeat that you will see Miracles through your hands through MINE. Conviction really comes through accomplishment. Remember that ability is the potential, Achievement is its expression, and Atonement is the Purpose."

Urtext, Chapter 1, Introduction to Miracles

God's Voice speaks to you all through the day.

"It is quite possible to listen to God's Voice all through the day without interrupting your regular activities in any way. The part of your mind in which truth abides is in constant communication with God, whether you are aware of it or not. It is the other part of your mind that functions in the world and obeys the world's laws. It is this part which is constantly distracted, disorganized, and highly uncertain.

The part that is listening to the Voice of God is calm, always at rest and wholly certain. It is really the only part there is. The other part is a wild illusion, frantic and distraught, but without reality of any kind. Try today not to listen to it. Try to identify with the part of your mind where stillness and peace reign forever. Try to hear God's Voice call to you lovingly, reminding you that your Creator has not forgotten His Son."

ACIM, Lesson 49, God's Voice speaks to me all through the day

Exercise #1:

Start to differentiate between the ego's voice and God's Voice.

When the ego speaks, it will leave you feeling distraught, disorganized and highly uncertain. Don't listen to this voice. Ignore it totally.

When God speaks, His Voice will leave you feeling calm, always at rest and certain. This voice will make you happy with excitement.

Exercise #2:

Get calm. Breathe. Listen, and then set aside 30 minutes to write in your journal. Write freely, fast and leisurely. You might even want to write on loose paper so you can throw these pages away when you are done.

"Listen in deep silence. Be very still and open your mind. Go past all the raucous shrieks and sick imaginings that cover your real thoughts and obscure your eternal link with God. Sink deep into the peace that waits for you beyond the frantic, riotous thoughts and sounds and sights of this insane world. You do not live there. We are trying to reach your real home. We are trying to reach the place where you are truly welcome. We are trying to reach God."

ACIM, Lesson 49, God's Voice speaks to me all through the day

Exercise #3:

Look at what you've written. Which parts are ego (your addiction that beats you up and tells you how horrible you are) and which parts are the Holy Spirit? Are there any hidden clues or revealed secrets for you?

Exercise #4:

Still the loud raucous voice that has been keeping you small. When such thoughts occur, quietly step back, look at them, and let them go.

Following is a beautiful prayer Jesus gives in *A Course in Miracles* for coming to listen to the Voice for God within.

Lesson 254

Let every voice but God's be still in me.

Father, today I would but hear Your Voice. In deepest silence I would come to You, to hear Your Voice and to receive Your Word. I have no prayer but this: I come to You to ask You for the truth. And truth is but Your Will, which I would share with You today.

Today we let no evil thoughts direct our words or actions. When such thoughts occur, we quietly step back and look at them, and then we let them go. We do not want what they would bring with them. And so we do not choose to keep them. They are silent now. And in the stillness, hallowed by His Love, God speaks to us and tells us of our Will, as we have chosen to remember Him.

Day 35

Abundance

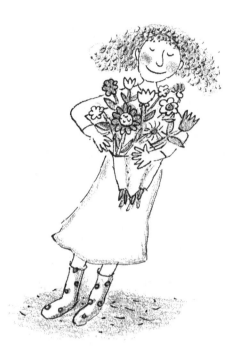

Abundance is a state of mind.

Marielle and I were originally going to call this topic MONEY but we realized that money is the wrong focus. When you focus on money (and your lack of it), you are coming from a place of limitation, which is obviously not abundance.

Praying for money is always going to result in you feeling like something is missing. It puts your focus on the future and the past. When you think about money there is an undercurrent of scarcity and lack.

The same goes for sickness. When you focus on your sickness, that's what you get.

When you begin changing your focus to what is going right (rather than on what is going wrong), you will witness dramatic miracles.

Abundance is the proper way of thinking. Abundance is now. Abundance focuses on all that you have.

Abundance is being in a state of gratitude and appreciation.

Abundance is luxuriating in life's simple pleasures.

To live in abundance is to live like royalty, no matter what your circumstances look like. Remember, abundance is a state of mind.

For five years I lived in a motel room which was part of church housing for a ministry program I was enrolled in. I had one room with a queen size bed, a beat-up couch, an old bureau, a night table with a lamp on it, a used desk, a bookshelf and a separate bathroom with a toilet, sink and bathtub.

For the first couple of years I was relatively neutral about my room. I felt neither gratitude nor grievance about it. It neither made me happy nor upset. I was traveling a lot those years (to New England, New York, Europe) and the room felt more like a storage area where I kept my stuff.

But then I started spending more time at home and I began to develop a grievance with the room. It was small and moldy. My closet was exposed and I started to get pissed off at my clothes for being out in plain sight. I had one small hot plate for cooking meals. I owned an electric water kettle for tea and coffee. I had a tiny refrigerator and I could never really see what was in it because the food was so cramped because of lack of space.

Lack. Limitation.

I did a lot of whining and complaining those years. I was angry at God a lot. I was angry at myself. I thought I deserved better.

Then a curious thing started happening: things started getting worse and worse and worse. I found myself in an absolute state of poverty. Most days I did not have a dollar to my name. I couldn't get a job. My debt was increasing. My gas tank was mostly on empty. I remember many times putting $2 worth of gas in my car (back when gas prices were $4/gallon)!

I spent all my time praying for money. I even tried manifesting money like the avatars I'd read about who could manifest money and objects out of thin air! I really truly believed that money would solve all my problems.

When I shopped for food I would buy the cheapest product possible. I only shopped at Wal-Mart. I wanted to do everything cheaply. Practically every fifth sentence out of my mouth was "I have no money."

My state of poverty was on my mind day and night!

One day I was complaining about my room to a friend and she started yelling at me: GET OVER YOURSELF LISA! YOU ARE SELFISH, BLIND AND UNGRATEFUL!

I was stunned. I was speechless.

She continued on with her yelling: YOU HAVE GOT TO START THINKING OF THAT ROOM AS A PALACE!

YOU HAVE GOT TO STOP SAYING "I HAVE NO MONEY!"

REMOVE THE PHRASE "I HAVE NO MONEY" FROM YOUR VOCABULARY!

She calmed down a little. She began to explain that I was holding myself in a state of limitation by constantly looking at what was wrong with my circumstances.

She said there was only one way out of poverty and that was through gratitude.

Gratitude, gratitude, gratitude.

She said that starting right then and there I was to think of myself as royalty and to start living my life as a magnificent Queen, realizing that I have everything.

She said my task was to begin living abundantly in a state of gratitude, no matter what my circumstances looked like.

If I felt pain, give thanks!
If I had a dollar, give thanks!
If I had a dime, give thanks!
When I met with a friend, give thanks!

Jesus tells us in *A Course in Miracles*:

"Only appreciation is an appropriate response to your brother."
Urtext, Chapter 11, The Judgment of the Holy Spirit

That day my life transformed. I've never known poverty since that day. When I walked into my room that afternoon it was truly like walking into a palace! I saw everything differently! The room was flooded with sunlight through my glass window that took up one whole wall. My cats, who had been lounging lazily and happily on the couch, went bananas in excitement that I was home. There was my desk! My beloved gorgeous desk! Such a "familiar place", a friend really! It was where I'd written hundreds of articles and my first book! And there was my closet! Oh, my closet! Look at my clothes! Beautiful fantastic stylish clothes, and shoes! Oh, the shoes! And here is my bed. Look at this bed! Beautiful! Stunning with a perfect white down comforter fit for a princess.

And books! Cherished and magnificent books!

The gratitude went on for about an hour, and never stopped. I kept finding new things to be grateful for in my room, which was now my palace.

At one point I hit an obstacle. I couldn't really be grateful for my bathroom with its cold tile floor and mold. But with a few cleaning supplies along with a can of white paint, white Christmas lights, a plush white rug, and tons of candles I turned my bathroom into a spa haven fit for a Princess!

Then I started finding other things to be grateful for in my life: my car, my friendships, my family, my successes, my failures, the sun shining in the sky, the rain, the snow, the wind.

I became so grateful for my room and for my life that I practically didn't notice that money was coming my way. The picture of my life began to change. Suddenly I was filling my gas tank to full every time I stopped at the gas station. My cupboards were filled with fabulous food. I was paying my bills. My relationships improved. My writing improved.

I had everything!

I'd always had everything, except that I was blind to it. I had been holding on to every little crumb and scrap, terrified and afraid, bemoaning my situation.

I laugh now because now I do physically live in a palace. I live in a 5-bedroom house with 2 kitchens, 3 living rooms, 3 hot tubs on 40 acres of land in the most beautiful scenic location I've ever seen in my life. My relationships are harmonious. I'm doing work I love.

Abundance.

The picture of my life changed because I changed.

<u>Exercise #1</u>

Be grateful. Make a gratitude list.

<u>Exercise #2:</u>

Shift your focus from poverty to abundance.

<u>Exercise #3:</u>

Realize that you have everything now.

<u>Exercise #4:</u>

See yourself as royalty and see your home as a palace.

WEEK 6
JOY

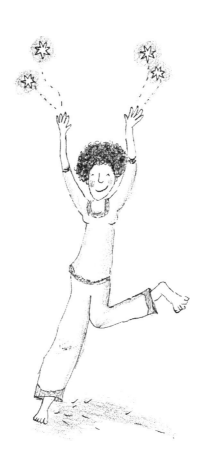

Day 36

Extension/Being in Love

Extension is the same as being in love.

When you are in love you are naturally extending light.

Do you want to know the most powerful way to let the light of you extend to others? I'm going to let you in on a little secret that will transform you and everyone around you.

Here it is: Be totally alert, present, and attentive with no judgment.

This might sound easy but very few people can actually do it.

Little children are masters at extension and being in love because they have nowhere else to be, other than the moment they are in.

If you get the opportunity to be with a small child, take advantage of it. A child is the perfect demonstration of how to extend. Simply spend an hour with him or her and watch the light move through the child to others.

Either borrow a child for an hour or go to Starbucks or the mall and sit quietly and observe children. You will be completely amazed.

They are in true extension. They don't give to get. They are purely themselves: joy, light, happiness and exuberant energy!

Watch other people's reaction to small children. The light of a small child affects everyone! It affects a person even if the child is all the way on the other side of the room! The light touches everyone. It shines through the child and transforms everyone.

Notice how erect a child's posture is. Little kids stand perfectly straight because their core is strong. Their center is powerful. Little kids don't slouch. Slouching comes later when the weight of the world starts crushing in on them.

Extension is about BEING PERFECTLY PRESENT IN THE MOMENT YOU ARE IN.

That's all! How simple!

The light does the work. As you step back, the light goes out from you and heals all things, including you.

"As you step back, the Light in you steps forward and encompasses the world."
      Urtext, Lesson 156, I walk with God in perfect holiness

Amazing! In extension, you don't do anything! You simply step back and the light in you steps forward.

"Healing is the result of using the body SOLELY for communication. Since this IS natural, it heals by making whole, which is also natural."
      Urtext, Chapter 8, Communication and the Ego-Body Equation

"When you equate yourself with a body, you will ALWAYS experience depression. When a Child of God thinks of himself in this way, he is belittling himself and seeing his brothers as similarly belittled. Since he can find himself ONLY in them, he has cut himself off from salvation. Remember that the Holy Spirit interprets the body ONLY as a means of communication. Being the communication link between God and His separated Sons, He interprets everything YOU have in the light of what HE is."
      Urtext, Chapter 8, Communication and the Ego-Body Equation

The ego SEPARATES through the body. The Holy Spirit reaches THROUGH it to others.

"The arrest of the mind's extension is the cause of illness."
ACIM Urtext, Chapter 8, Communication and the Ego-Body Equation

There are only two possible actions in every moment for you: extension or projection. Either you are EXTENDING the love that you are or you are PROJECTING a world because you think you are a body and you think your brother is a body.

There is nothing between these two choices.

Either you are in extension of love or you are in judgment. Either you are giving in joy or you are feeling guilty. Either you are in full creation and extension or you are in a black hole, depressed.

Either you are extending in light or you're turning in on yourself.

This is the range. You are in Heaven or hell, and there is no in-between.

Here are words from Jesus in *A Course in Miracles*:

"When you look upon a brother as a physical entity, his power and glory are lost to you and SO ARE YOURS. You have attacked him and you must have attacked yourself first. Do not see him this way for your own salvation, which MUST bring him his. Do not ALLOW him to belittle himself in your mind, but give him freedom from his belief in littleness, and escape from yours. As part of YOU, he is holy. As part of ME, you are. To communicate with a part of God Himself is to reach beyond the Kingdom to its Creator, through His Voice which He has established as part of you.

"Mind cannot be made physical, but it can be made manifest THROUGH the physical if it uses the body to GO BEYOND itself. By reaching out, the mind EXTENDS itself. It does not stop at the body, for if it does it is blocked in its purpose. A mind which has been blocked has allowed itself to be vulnerable to attack, because it has TURNED AGAINST ITSELF."
Urtext, Chapter 8, Communication and the Ego-Body Equation

YOU ARE PERFECT AS GOD CREATED YOU.

Perfect!

The only thing that needs to be changed is your own thinking. When you gut out the black spot in your thinking, your body will transform all by itself.

Forget about trying to change your body! Forget about dieting! Forget about exercise to get in shape! All that is needed is that you become vigilant to change your thinking.

YOU ARE ALL LIGHT.

There will be temptations along the way from yourself and others. You will have moments when you think you are ugly and despicable. You will feel grossly distorted. People will give you all sorts of advice.

Here is the only advice you'll ever really need:

"YOUR BODY IS A MEANS OF COMMUNICATION."

"ONLY APPRECIATION IS AN APPROPRIATE RESPONSE TO A BROTHER."

"The opposite of joy is depression. When your learning promotes depression instead of joy, you cannot be listening to God's joyous Teacher, and you must be learning amiss. To see a body as anything EXCEPT a means of pure extension is to limit your mind and hurt yourself. Health is therefore nothing more than united purpose. If the body is brought under the purpose of the mind, it becomes whole because mind's purpose is one."
Urtext, Chapter 8, Communication and the Ego-Body Equation

The power of wholeness is EXTENSION.

"Do not arrest your thought in this world, and you will open your mind to Creation in God."
Urtext, Chapter 8, Communication and the Ego-Body Equation

What does all this mean??? What does it mean to extend?

Extension is pure awareness of yourself as whole, complete and perfect. In your pure awareness of yourself as light, love, joy and happiness you see everyone else as light, love, joy and happiness. That's extension.

EXTENSION IS PURE PRESENCE.

The light extends. Your body doesn't do anything.

To extend is to be in a condition of non-judgment. It is to see yourself and your brothers as pure light.

Extension is to look beyond the body.

Addicts identify almost exclusively with the body. Practically everything they do is wrapped up in bodies, appearances and trying to improve their condition (and improve the condition of people around them through advice).

Exercise #1:

Think of yourself as precious.

If you do only one thing in this 40-day course, let it be this exercise. You are a precious child of God. Never forget it.

Exercise #2:

Stop trying to improve yourself and other people. Let everything be exactly as it is.

Exercise #3:

Practice non-judgment. Let everything be exactly as it is.

Exercise #4:

Fall deeply and madly in love with yourself.

List all the qualities you like about yourself. These attributes can include innocence, purity, generosity, kindness, gentleness, commitment, dedication, honoring your word, open-mindedness, honesty, patience, joy.

Realize how awesomely magnificent you truly are!

Exercise #5:

Fall deeply and madly in love with everyone you see.

Recognize your brother's incredible attributes: innocence, purity, generosity, kindness, gentleness, commitment, dedication, honoring his/her word, open-mindedness, honesty, patience, joy.

You are royalty.

Your brother is royalty.

Day 37

Laughter

Laughter is the best medicine.

This is a fact.

HERE ARE THE HEALTH BENEFITS OF LAUGHTER:

Laughter boosts levels of endorphins.
Laughter reduces pain.
Laughter improves flow of oxygen.
Laughter decreases stress levels.
Laughter strengthens your immune system.
Laughter is good for your heart.
Laughter improves the function of blood cells and increases blood flow.
Laughter relaxes your muscles.
Laughter increases your energy.

A tremendous amount of healing comes from laughter.

At the most basic level: LAUGHTER MAKES YOU FEEL GOOD!

For most addicts, laughter does not come naturally. Addicts tend to be serious about everything. They've taught themselves about "responsibility" and about the importance of "keeping up appearances."

Laughter – real laughter – changes you.

Scientific studies have shown that laughter has significant, positive effects on the body. So, perhaps the best "exercise" you can do for yourself is laugh.

Exercise #1:

Write down all the things that make you laugh.

Exercise #2:

Laugh.

Make it a priority to laugh every day.

Easier said than done, right??? How can someone who has been trapped in addiction, sickness or depression start laughing on a daily basis?

When you realize the importance of laughter, you will find a way!

Children, movies, books, and animals are a treasure house for funny moments.

Exercise #3:

Call a friend (or invite one out for coffee or a movie) with the single intention of having a good time and laughing together.

"Into eternity, where all is one, there crept a tiny mad idea, at which the Son of God remembered not to laugh. In his forgetting did the thought become a serious idea, and possible of both accomplishment and real effects. Together, we can laugh them BOTH away, and understand that time can NOT intrude upon eternity. It IS a joke to think that time can come to circumvent eternity, which MEANS there is no time."
Urtext, Chapter 27, The 'Hero' of the Dream

Day 38

Physical Healing/Transformation

We are almost at the end of our 40-day trek into the Wilderness with Jesus.

I love how my friend Marjukka described these 40-days. She called them "her honeymoon with Jesus."

Yes!

Marielle and I promised you that you'd be healed of food addiction in 40 days and we meant it. This journey is about physical healing and transformation.

For myself, I am amazed how truly different I became in only 40 days.

When I first started my "40 days", I was confronted by the devil (in the form of a good friend who asked me when I was going to start losing weight). It was a strange episode. I was happy and joyful, and feeling more beautiful than I'd ever felt in my entire life, and we were having fun together. Then out of nowhere this friend started pointing out all that he saw as physically wrong with me: my stomach, my thighs, my butt. He said he thought I should be running with the dogs every day instead of just having fun with them and taking them for long walks. Usually I'd accept these kinds of words as "fact" and then eat a box of cookies once I'm home alone.

But this time, I got mad!

I said: WHAT?!?! WHO ARE YOU?? WHAT KIND OF NONSENSE IS THIS? ARE YOU LISTENING TO WHAT YOU ARE SAYING? WHO ARE YOU?

He said he was trying to be helpful. He said he thought I wanted to do something about my weight.

Oh my God!

I was mad! I kept yelling. I told him I was happier and felt more beautiful than ever in my entire life.

I yelled for five minutes straight. It felt like exorcising demons.

It was healing and transforming. I'd never stood up for myself before in quite that way. I made a huge loud scene. I felt gorgeous! I felt strong and powerful! I never protected the Christ-child in me with such force and care.

Physical transformation is often really messy.

You're slaying dragons. Transformation can be terrifying and lonely. You're out there in the desert of your mind confronted by the "enemy", which is *you*. You're hacking out destructive habits and old beliefs that no longer serve you. There's blood, guts and gore. You can end up feeling exhausted because you are truly in a battle with demons (all your own thoughts) that are determined to keep you small and limited.

I read a great quote this week:

"Everything you really want is just outside your comfort zone."
–Robert Allen

My comfort zone lies in staying small and quiet; in being the good girl who never rocks the boat.

Everything I want is outside of that zone.

When I stood up for my innocence and beauty, I was outside of my comfort zone.

But afterward, I felt completely different! I entered a whole new segment of life. The past was gone. How wild! I woke up the next morning a completely different person! Usually I would feel guilty for "sleeping in" (which is any time after 5am). And since practically every day I would sleep past 5am, I pretty much felt guilty every day. Amazing, huh? Making myself feel guilty before the sun even rises and before my feet even touch the floor! LOL. Then I'd race out of bed in a frantic dash and immediately turn on the computer to write the daily blog entries. Rush! Rush! Rush! I'm late! I'm late! I'm late!

But after having stood up for myself with this friend, it was like the Queen of England woke up in my body! I had no cares and no worries. I knew instinctively that everything would happen perfectly in its own way, in its own time. I woke up at 5am the next morning, feeling all luxurious and comfy in my bed, incredibly happy, without any trace of guilt.

You often cannot see how dramatically your life has shifted from the point you are standing in. Only when you look back and compare THEN versus NOW can you begin to see the changes in yourself.

Only one exercise for today, and it's a good one:

Exercise #1:

List all things that are different in your life since you started this 40-day program.

Following is my list as it occurred for me. On my 38th day, I wrote:

I complete projects.
I take care of myself.
I ask for help.
I dusted off the juicer and I use it.
I bought a bike and ride it almost every day.
I started a radio show.
I got a camera and am becoming an amateur photographer.
I spend half my day playing and having fun.

I don't worry about anything anymore.

I feel truly gorgeous, physically beautiful. This is a miracle.

I got new contact lenses and even splurged on a new pair of glasses! (I'd been putting off the doctor appointment for contact lenses for a year! And the last time I bought new glasses was 15 years ago)

I am paying my debts. Another huge miracle!

I know that everything I want, I'm going to receive exactly as I ask for it.

I feel happy when I eat instead of feeling guilty. Another dramatic miracle!

I feel excited when I wake up in the morning.

Day 39

Happiness

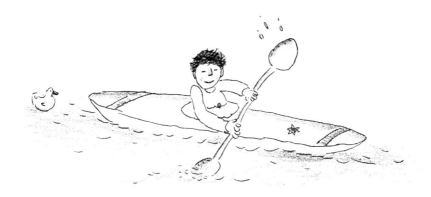

You only need to choose for your happiness once to have it forever.

Happiness is not elusive.

Happiness is not fleeting.

Happiness is not based on external events, people or situations happening outside of you.

Happiness is an INTERNAL-ETERNAL STATE OF MIND that you choose for yourself. Happiness is a gift that you give to yourself.

You can have anything you want! Happiness is your decision. Happiness is CONSTANT once you decide that it is your goal.

Happiness is a self-taught ability to be deeply affected by love!

A Course in Miracles asks "Do you want to be right or do you want to be happy?"

Trust me when I tell you that chaos will continue as always. People are still going to be demanding your attention. They might attack you. They might say mean things to you. But you – YOU! – who have chosen for happiness will remain completely unaffected by the storm that is swirling around you.

This world is a place of madness. According to *A Course in Miracles*, the world is a "slaughterhouse." Problems are not fixable. Relationships are not fixable. So stop wasting your time and energy trying to change people and events so that it suits you.

The only thing you really need to focus on is your own happiness.

Does this sound selfish to you?
God's Will for you is perfect happiness!

It's your will to be happy. It's not selfish. It's the most natural thing in the world. It's God's Will for you!

Now, here is an interesting fact: "Guilt creeps in where happiness has been removed and SUBSTITUTES for it."
Urtext, Chapter 19, The Attraction of Guilt

Isn't that interesting??? *When you are not happy, it is guaranteed you are experiencing guilt.* When I am not happy and joyous, I always feel like I should be doing something to improve myself or my situation. Guilt, Guilt, Guilt. I feel like I should "fix" something. Guilty as charged.

But when I am happy, I am in the NOW. I am present, knowing that everything is perfect! When I am happy and at peace I feel like I am exactly where I am supposed to be, right where I am now. I am relaxed and content, trusting, knowing, and rejoicing.

"The Holy Spirit needs a happy learner in whom His mission can be happily accomplished."
ACIM, Chapter 14, The Happy Learner

As you enter into a state of happiness, you enter into what Jesus calls "The Happy Dream."

Happiness occurs by your decision. Happiness is not going to be given to you on a silver platter. You must decide for it and make it your overriding choice in every situation all through the day. Believe me, everything and everyone in time and space is designed to distract you! Everything! This is called "mind-training" for a reason. You have to continually keep catching your thoughts and bringing yourself back gently to your goal: HAPPINESS.

True Happiness means you are no longer affected by anything outside of you. Nothing has power over you anymore. Nothing has the ability to make you happy or sad. It's all you! How wonderful!

You don't have to wait for someone to send you roses or to tell you he loves you. YOU KNOW YOU'RE LOVED! You stop needing confirmation from other people. It's nice when it arrives, but you no longer need it. Your happiness no longer depends on the world.

You're suddenly happy for no reason at all! You're happy because your life is an adventure! You're happy because you've located the source of all creativity and power: in your own mind! You've tapped into a treasure house that belongs to you! You're happy because now you KNOW that you create your own reality!

You're happy because you realize how very powerful you truly are. You begin to realize your grace, beauty, innocence, purity and strength.

Exercise #1:

Write down what makes you happy.

What makes your heart sing? What feels effortless, like playing, when you do it?

<u>Exercise #2:</u>

Imagine the most perfect life for yourself. This is The Happy Dream. Write down a detailed specific description of The Happy Dream and how it looks for you. This is your dream.

WHAT DO YOU WANT?

What do you do for work? What kinds of experiences do you have? What are your relationships like? What kind of clothes do you wear? What does your day look like? Where do you shop? What kind of foods do you eat? Do you travel? Where do you go? What kind of house do you live in? What time do you wake up in the morning? What time do you go to bed? What are your hobbies? What do you do for fun?

Day 40

Function/Purpose

It is your function to accept yourself as God created you... perfect.

You are perfect right in this moment, exactly the way you are and you do not need to change anything. You are healed, whole and perfect, shining in the reflection of God's Love.

YOU ARE A MASTERPIECE!

"Your function is not little."
ACIM, Chapter 15, Littleness versus Magnitude

"You who are now the bringer of salvation have the function of bringing light to darkness. The darkness in you has been brought to light. Carry it back to darkness, from the holy instant to which you brought it. We are made whole in our desire to make whole."
ACIM, Chapter 18, Light in the Dream

Here are a few facts:
You are all light. You are pure innocence, grace, purity, and beauty. You are creative and all-powerful.

You are Spirit, a light that is brighter than the sun that lights the sky, with a Friend Who goes with you wherever you go.

Your function is to remember how gorgeous you are! How simple! And when you forget, your function is to forgive yourself.

Be gentle with yourself. When you forget your Identity in God, simply dust yourself off, and get back in alignment as quickly as possible.

That's your function. It's not complicated. Your function is to be happy.

It's time to do what you love to do. It's time to find out what you want.

Your function is NOT to knock yourself out trying to be everywhere at once. Your function is NOT about overwhelming yourself, pretending to be bright and happy when you simply need to rest. Your function is NOT to exhaust yourself through constant giving, helping, teaching.

Remember, there is no world. There are no other people. There is only you.

Your function is to remember your perfection and innocence. You are a Child of God, and your function is to continually align yourself with this vibration of Love.

"O my child, if you knew what God wills for you, your joy would be complete! And what He wills has happened, for it was always true. When the light comes and you have said, 'God's Will is mine,' you will see such beauty that you will know it is not of you. Out of your joy you will create beauty in His Name, for your joy could no more be contained than His."

ACIM, Chapter 11, From Darkness to Light

<u>Exercise #1:</u>

Accept your function as God's greatest gift to the world. YOU ARE A MASTERPIECE. You are all light. *It is your function to be happy.*

<u>Exercise #2:</u>

Relate to yourself as Spirit. Find that place in you where you are free from addiction.

Here is one more gift that came my way yesterday.

These are the words of Abraham-Hicks, from the book *The Law of Attraction: The Basics of the Teachings of Abraham.* Jerry & Esther

Hicks have published over 800 Abraham-Hicks books, cassettes, CDs, and DVDs and their work is beautiful, practical and life-changing. You can find more information at their website: http://www.abraham-hicks.com

I hope these words inspire you if you are still not convinced of your healing. If you are not getting the results you had hoped for in this 40-day program and if you are impatient to see progress, I pray these words will be helpful to you:

Abraham:
"When you are clear about everything you want, you will get all the results that you want. But often you are not completely clear. You say for example, 'I want the color yellow and I want the color blue' but what you end up with is the color green. And then you say 'How did I get green? I did not intend that at all.' But it came forth as a blending of other intentions, you see. Blending the color yellow with blue creates the color green.

In a similar manner (at an unconscious level) there is a blending of intentions that is continually occurring within you, but it is so complex that your conscious thinking mechanism cannot sort it out. But your Inner Being can sort it out, and can offer you guiding emotions. All that is required is that you pay attention to the way you feel, and that you let yourself be drawn to those things that feel good or right *to you* while you let yourself be moved away from those things that do not."

Epilogue

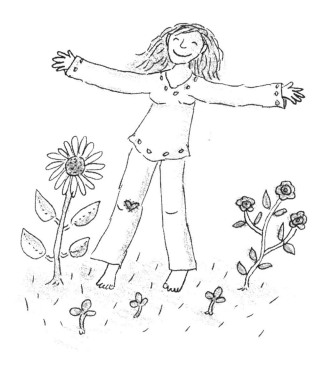

You are whole and perfect as God created you.

This is not the end but the beginning. You will probably still have days when you slide back into old patterns: patterns of guilt, shame, uncertainty, and eating everything but the kitchen sink. That's okay.

What we have found is that the amount of time that you hold on to guilt or shame gets shorter and shorter. You catch yourself more quickly. Where before you might have felt horrible for weeks (or years) because you thought your body wasn't perfect, now you might only feel it for an hour before remembering one of the lessons from this book. Suddenly you realize you really ARE doing things differently. Instead of sitting alone and eating a box of cookies, you call a friend. Instead of drowning your sorrows in ice cream, you take a bubble bath. Suddenly, there comes that magical moment when you realize you're not thinking about food all day long. It's a miracle! This usually comes as an unexpected surprise when it occurs to you that you are at last *living* your life, and not obsessing/thinking about food anymore. You eat when you're hungry. What a miracle!

It Matters Totally is a spiritual journey back to the remembrance of your true Self as God created you. If you need help, you can find mighty companions at our website http://www.itmatterstotally.com

We also suggest, if you have not done so already, to get a copy of *A Course in Miracles*. It's a beautiful book. It's a love letter from Jesus to you.

Remember, you are not alone. All the help you need is available. All you have to do is ask for it.

Here is the best advice that was ever given to me and now I give it to you: Have fun.

Love, Lisa

A final note from Marielle:

Dear reader,

At this point of the book you might be very happy or very disappointed or somewhere in between.

You might be excited with the changes that have occurred in you, or you might be feeling: this is not working for me.

Whatever emotions you are experiencing, I would like you to know, "It is okay." It is not necessary to feel that anything should be different. Your healing needs to be given, and that is all there is to it. Whenever you feel you suffer from self-hatred or judgment, or you can't stop being mean to yourself, contact us. We can be your strength and your love for a moment. That is how it was given to me: in my weakness, not in my strength, and in my total inability to be or to have the solution. I learned to reach out to others and ask for help.

Your healing doesn't have to look a certain way. It will be all yours. *Very unique.* It took me a long time to realize that all I needed was communication. It was important for me to find my own expression.

I love you for going through this 40-day journey. Thank you. I AM HERE FOR YOU. You are amazing and very free. It might seem difficult for a moment, but remember ... you are not alone. You can connect with others who are going through the same experiences.

A life long habit in which you have denied yourself everything is powerful and often overwhelming. If you remember that fact, and know that you don't have to fix it, you won't be discouraged. You will know the fall-backs are part of the healing. It will make you stronger.

IT IS ABOUT LITTLE CHANGES - ALWAYS!

It used to shock me as I learned that I could be joyful and supportive of myself. Until it felt like ME. Every little thing that I did for myself was helpful. And it changed my genetic memory. It really works.

I hope to meet you at our web-site.
Please stay in touch.

Loving you,
Marielle

CPSIA information can be obtained at www.ICGtesting.com
Printed in the USA
LVOW091847281011

252554LV00027B/77/P